I0791339

# What Others Say

Victor Shane in *Millennial Medicine* presents a strong and detailed argument that the attack on the plague of cancer should be aimed at what many believe is its root cause: the malfunctioning of the cell's repair mechanism, the mitochondria. Shane then associates this malfunctioning as due to the mitochondria receiving malnutrition, the junk foods and processed foods that we feed it. An interesting nuance in the search for a cure.

—Gerald L. Schroeder, PhD
Jerusalem, Israel


In his wide-ranging book, Shane skillfully points out the mounting empirical evidence that modern nutritional deficits may contribute to cancer and clearly offers some valuable advice about healthy eating and lifestyles.

—Kirkus Reviews

Other books by Victor Shane

*The Church in Eclipse: Restoring the Light*

*The Authentic Life*
A Guidebook for Millennials: Preparing the Next Generation to Lead

*Millennial Economics*
An American Declaration of Independence from Central Banking: The Global Transition to Debt-Free National Economics

*In God We Trust*
Understanding the Culture War in a Scientific Age: The Pitched Battle for the Soul of America

*Book of Life*
God, Cosmos and Man: A New Understanding of Human Nature: A Holistic Defense of the Judeo-Christian Ethic

# MILLENNIAL MEDICINE

## CRITICAL PATH TO ROOTING OUT CANCER IN TWENTY-FIVE YEARS

Victor Shane

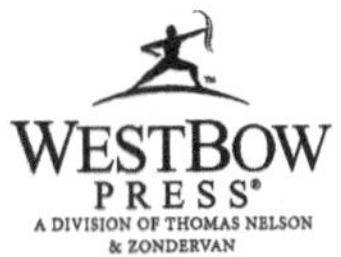

WESTBOW
PRESS®
A DIVISION OF THOMAS NELSON
& ZONDERVAN

WestBow Press books may be ordered through booksellers or by contacting:

WestBow Press
A Division of Thomas Nelson & Zondervan
1663 Liberty Drive
Bloomington, IN 47403
www.westbowpress.com
844-714-3454



ISBN: 978-1-6642-7054-1 (sc)
ISBN: 978-1-6642-7055-8 (hc)
ISBN: 978-1-6642-7056-5 (e)

Library of Congress Control Number: 2022911862

Print information available on the last page.

WestBow Press rev. date: 7/23/2022

## Disclaimer

The information, content, and ideas expressed in this book are the opinions of its author and are not to be construed as medical advice. Neither the author nor the publisher shall be liable or responsible for any loss or damage or injury allegedly arising from any information, content, idea, or opinion published in this book. Always seek the advice of your physician or qualified health care provider with any questions that you may have regarding a medical condition.

Let food be thy medicine and medicine be thy food.

—Hippocrates (circa 400 BC)

Maintaining a strong and healthy body are prerequisites to serving God! After all, one who is ill cannot possibly devote his energy and focus to the study of his Creator. Thus, it is a legal obligation to refrain from all items that harm your health. It is equally a legal obligation to discipline yourself in all habits that strengthen and invigorate your body.

—Rabbi Moses Ben Maimon (Maimonides)
Mishneh Torah, *Hilchot Deot*,
Chapter 4 (circa AD 1170)

# Contents

# Foreword

It is a pleasure for me to write the foreword to Victor Shane's important book on the current cancer crisis, *Millennial Medicine*. Unless there is a paradigm shift in treatment and prevention strategies, cancer will soon overtake heart disease as the leading cause of suffering and death in Western societies. Our evaluation of data from the American Cancer Society showed that the number of people dying in the US from cancer in 2013 was 580,350, and in 2020, it was 606,520, an increase of 4.3 percent. In other words, over 1,600 people are dying from cancer each day in the US. The US population increase over this same period was about 4.5 percent, indicating no real progress in cancer management despite the continuous hype surrounding new drugs and radiation treatments. Indeed, some new immunotherapy drugs can cause "hyperprogressive" disease, or the lethal acceleration of tumor growth. As long as cancer is considered a genetic disease, there will be little or no changes in the current standards of care.

Emerging evidence indicates that the failure to reduce the number deaths from cancer has been due to an incorrect theory on the origin of the disease. We recently provided extensive evidence showing that the genetic or somatic mutation theory, which has driven basic cancer research and drug development for decades, is no longer credible. Drug development based on a flawed theory will produce ineffective drugs with unacceptable toxicities. We clearly described how the mitochondrial metabolic theory can explain better the origin of cancer than can the somatic mutation theory (Seyfried and Chinopoulos, *Metabolites*, 2021). The recognition of cancer as a metabolic disease now justifies the use of novel nontoxic, costeffective therapeutic strategies for both managing and preventing cancer. *Millennial Medicine* calls out to the millennial generation in layman's terms the paradigm shift that will be necessary for reversing the trend of increasingly more people suffering relentlessly and dying from cancer.

The simple definition of *cancer* is "cell division out of control." Cancer is a systemic disturbance in the body involving multiple time- and space-dependent changes in the health status of cells and tissues that ultimately lead to malignant tumors. Chronic damage to mitochondria-regulated energy metabolism will eventually cause normal cells to grow out of control and become malignant. It is the mitochondria in the cytoplasm of our cells that maintains the state of quiescent differentiation and regulated growth. The mitochondria control the energy homeostasis of our cells and ultimately that of our entire body through the process of oxidative phosphorylation (OxPhos), i.e., energy from breathing oxygen. The carbons from the food we eat are combined in the mitochondria with the oxygen that we breathe to form the energy of life. This respiratory energy production is highly efficient in maintaining regulated cell growth. The waste products of OxPhos are water and carbon dioxide, much of which is released in our breath.

Cancer involves chronic damage to the number, structure, and function of mitochondria in cells of our organs. This damage can arise from diet and lifestyle issues together with broad range of risk factors, including radiation exposure, chronic inflammation, intermittent hypoxia, chemical carcinogens, rare inherited mutations, oncogenic viruses, and advancing age. Abnormalities to mitochondrial integrity within a cell will gradually disrupt energy production through OxPhos, causing the cell to compensate by increasing energy production through the ancient pathways of fermentation.

Fermentation involves energy production in the absence of oxygen. Fermentation was the predominant mechanism for energy production in all cells prior to the emergence of oxygen in earth's atmosphere some 2.5 billion years ago. Unbridled cell proliferation characterized most of the cells living at that time. These primitive cells would proliferate as long as they had access to fermentable fuels in their environment.

Energy production from fermentation, however, is highly inefficient. Large amounts of fermentable fuels are required in the extracellular environment to drive energy production through fermentation. Fermentation is also the mechanism for energy generation in all major cancers, including those of the breast, colon, lung, brain, liver, kidney, ovary, bladder, pancreas, bone, and prostate. Simply stated, fermentation metabolism is the driving force for all major cancers. Unlike normal cells that use OxPhos for energy production, cancer cells are dependent on fermentation for energy production. The sugar glucose and the amino acid glutamine are the two major fuels necessary for driving the fermentation metabolism of all growing cancers. The higher the blood sugar, the faster is the tumor growth, whereas the lower the blood sugar, the slower is the tumor growth. Unfortunately, the linkage of high blood sugar to rapid cancer growth remains unknown to most laypeople and oncologists, as some cancer patients are often given, and readily accept, high-carbohydrate drinks and foods during their treatments.

In contrast to normal cells that produce water and carbon dioxide as waste products, cancer cells produce large amounts of lactic acid as a waste product of their fermentation metabolism. Oxidative stress from defective respiration, together with lactic acid dumping into the tumor microenvironment, causes the genetic abnormalities observed in the nucleus of the cancer cells. In other words, the mutations observed in the tumor cells are not the cause of cancer but are downstream effects of the abnormal energy metabolism. This can explain in large part why cancer drug development based on the genetic theory produces ineffective drugs. Moreover, the dumping of cancer fermentation waste products causes acidification of the microenvironment, leading to metastasis, or the spread of cancer cells throughout the body. The management and eventual resolution of cancer will thus involve therapies that can effectively restrict fermentable fuels (glucose and glutamine) to the tumor cells while transitioning the body to nonfermentable fuels (ketone bodies), which the tumor cells cannot use for energy. Unfortunately, the cancer academic and pharmaceutical industries either do not know about this information or choose to ignore it.

*Millennial Medicine* outlines a clear path for preventing cancer and for simplifying the treatment and business models currently used for managing cancer. If the current path is not changed, the millennial generation will bear the manifold effects of both the physical and financial toxicities associated with cancer. As long as cancer is viewed as a genetic disease, there will be no major improvements in survival rates. The current path can be reversed, however, if those diagnosed with cancer can ask their oncologists a few simple questions:

> First, is my treatment strategy based on the genetic or the metabolic theory of cancer?
> Second, how will my planned treatment strategy be able to restrict glucose and glutamine to my tumor?
> Finally, how effective will your ketogenic metabolic dietary plan be in improving my overall health during the treatment?

Credible answers to these questions will require some level of scientific literacy on the part of both the patient and the oncologist. The general concepts presented in *Millennial Medicine* provide a road map to help those diagnosed with cancer to improve their quality of life and overall chances for survival.

Thomas N. Seyfried, PhD
Professor of Biology, Boston College
Author of *Cancer as a Metabolic Disease: On the Origin, Management, and Prevention of Cancer*

# Author's Introduction

Attention, millennials: before you know it, the previous generation will pass away, and you will inherit the health-care mess they leave behind. How will you deal with the challenges you are about to face in that regard? How will history judge you? Will history say, "The millennials came and went, and nothing changed—there is more diabetes, more heart disease, more cancer!"?

The author is persuaded that history will render a better judgment of you and has written a number of books to inspire you to pursue the high roads that lead to the auspicious plateaus of liberty, prosperity, and vigorous health. Speaking of vigorous health, one of the challenges that you will shortly face relates to the plague of the twentieth century: cancer. And this is where you will have to roll up your sleeves and "go to war," so to speak, not so much with the devil of cancer itself, but with the deeply entrenched errors of twentieth-century medicine.

Not to worry; time is on your side. As the great physicist Max Planck once remarked:

> A new scientific truth does not triumph by convincing
> its opponents and making them see the light, but rather
> because its opponents eventually die, and a new generation
> grows up that is familiar with it.

You are that new generation. With God's help, you will succeed in making the world a cancer-free place for all the families of the earth to live and prosper in. You can do it, but bear in mind that time is the greatest thief of them all. Time doesn't stand still for anyone—alas, not even for you! *Tempus fugit, igitur carpe diem!*

# *Chapter 1*

# Cancer

To know your enemy, you must become your enemy.
—Sun Tzu, *The Art of War,* 490 BC

President Nixon declared war on cancer back in 1971. Fifty years later, hundreds of thousands of Americans continue to die of the disease every year. Last year, it was around six hundred thousand, and the number has been more or the less the same year after year. Men, women, young, old, rich, poor, Black, White, Asian, Hispanic, Jewish, gentile, friends, brothers, sisters, fathers, mothers, uncles, aunts, grandfathers, and grandmothers keep dying of cancer, and we seem unable to do anything about it. How does this happen? What are we going to do about it? What are we going to do about this affront to our human dignity? What are we going to do about this violation of our God-given right to life?

Maybe the reason we are losing the battle against cancer is because we really don't know what it is that we are fighting. It seems we've been chasing our own tails, shadowboxing, grasping at straws, trying this and that, throwing billions of dollars at a spot on the wall and then painting a target around it. You can't win the war against cancer this way. To win the war, you must come to know your enemy firsthand. As the Chinese general Sun Tzu once said, "To know your enemy, you must become your enemy."

## The Philosophy of Cancer

Before we waste billions more dollars doing the same thing and expecting a different result (which is Einstein's definition of insanity, by the way), we must make a serious effort to come to know our enemy intimately. What is this devil called cancer all about? What's it up to? What does it want from us? Start with the most basic of philosophical questions: Is this devil Manichaean or Augustinian? Is it a clever fiend who's trying to do us in, or is it the outworking of some universal principle that to this day eludes our apprehension? Mathematician and philosopher Norbert Weiner (1894-1964) tackled a similar question decades ago:

> The scientist is always working to discover the order and organization of the universe, and is thus playing a game against the arch enemy, disorganization. Is this devil Manichaean or Augustinian? Is it a contrary force opposed to order or is it the very absence of order itself? The difference between these two sorts of demons will make itself apparent in the tactics to be used against them.[1]

Compare Weiner's remarks with the following by Travis Christofferson in his book, *Tripping Over the Truth*:

> Whether God, Mother Nature, evolution, or whatever shaped the world we live in, we must concede that in the realm of disease, cancer is her masterpiece. It is the Bobby Fischer, the George Patton, the Mozart, the Houdini, and Einstein of maladies. The way she has enticed us with comprehension only to pull back out of our reach is horrible, and, I dare say, even beautiful. Cancer is pathological artistry. Even Sherlock Holmes respected the master criminal he could not catch.[2]

While we would prefer to avoid the topics of devil and religion altogether, the answer to the philosophical question is germane because, as Wiener points out, it will determine the tactic to be used against it. A

---

[1] Norbert Wiener, *The Human Use of Human Beings* (New York, Da Capo Press, Inc. 1954), 34–36.

[2] Travis Christofferson, *Tripping Over the Truth* (White River Junction: Chelsea Green Publishing, 2017), 182.

Manichaean devil would likely be found in a chaotic universe in which anything goes, in which case we might as well learn to live with cancer. An Augustinian devil, on the other hand, would likely be found in a rational universe whose ontology we do not yet fully understand—in which case we need to go back to the drawing board and get our science straight. Check.

## Otto Warburg

When it comes to the history of cancer, the name that always comes up is that of German scientist and Nobel laureate Otto Heinrich Warburg (1883–1970). It seems, however, that even Warburg was somewhat off the mark, as his student and colleague, Nobel laureate Hans Krebs (after whom the "Krebs cycle" is named), suggests:

> Warburg neglected the fundamental biochemical aspect of the cancer problem, that of the mechanisms which are responsible for the uncontrolled growth of normal cells and which are lost or disturbed in the cancer cell. No doubt, the difference in energy metabolism discovered by Warburg are important, but however important, they are at a level of biochemical organization of the cell, not deep enough to touch the heart of the cancer problem, the uncontrolled growth.[3]

## Vogelstein's Resort to "Dark Matter"

Allow me to digress for a moment. In order to accelerate your car, you must press on the gas pedal (apply additional energy). The same principle holds in cosmology. In order to accelerate the expansion of the universe (presently thought to be the case), you would need additional energy. Meaning what? Meaning the quantity of energy in the universe is increasing? Impossible!

---

[3] Hans Krebs, *Otto Warburg, Cell Physiologist, Biochemist, and Eccentric* (First published in German in 1979, translated into English and published in 1981, reprinted in 2019 by Ishi Press International, New York and Tokyo, with a new introduction by Sam Sloan), 25–26.

So, then, where is the additional energy coming from? Could it be coming from some hitherto unknown "dark source"?

With the advent of the Human Genome Project in 1990 and the Cancer Genome Atlas in 2005, it was thought that scientists would finally be in a position to identify the mutation(s) responsible for the initiation of cancer. That was not to be the case, however. The cancer riddle was not solved at that time. The extent to which the riddle keeps evading the best minds of science is evident in researcher Bert Vogelstein's resort to "dark matter." As Christofferson relates:

> Vogelstein borrowed the term *dark matter* from astrophysics and applied it to the gaping hole in understanding revealed by the TCGA [*The Cancer Genome Atlas*]. He was aware that some nebulous, presumptive process was driving cancer. It was preventing the complete picture of cancer from being realized.[4]

## The Logic behind the Facts

One of the basic mandates of science is to discover "the logic behind the facts." When it comes to the devil of cancer, however, the logic seems to be missing. What is the logic, for example, behind the fact that at a certain point, the human body will go out of its way to sidestep its own defenses, tippy-toe around its own robust immune arsenals, and bend over backward to build a network of brand-new blood vessels around tumors so they can grow faster and metastasize? Where is the logic behind this maddening fact?

Call it "devil," call it "dark matter," call it "some nebulous, presumptive process," call it Alfred Hitchcock's "MacGuffin," or call it Monty Python's "blancmange," the fact is that something big is missing in cancer's picture, something that we must expose to the light of science if we are to win the war against the insidious disease. Christofferson states:

---

[4] Travis Christofferson, *Tripping Over the Truth* (White River Junction: Chelsea Green Publishing, 2017), 115.

Cancer stands alone as our most ardent, confusing, shape-shifting, and devastating enemy. The numbers don't lie. This year, almost six hundred thousand Americans will die from cancer ... Despite embellished announcements from government actuaries, the real death rates from cancer are the same today as they were in the 1950s. We can't seem to penetrate its elusive armor, and it's not for lack of trying ... Maybe the reason for the stunted progress goes far deeper than we thought. Maybe it is fundamental, going all the way [down] to the scientific bedrock at the true heart of the disease.[5]

To win the war against cancer, we must take the journey all the way down to what Christofferson calls "the scientific bedrock at the true heart of the disease." We must put on the training wheels, go back to school, and review the very first principles of science. Fasten your seat belts!

_________________

[5] *ibid,* "In the Beginning" (opening comments), xxi

## Chapter 2

# The Scientific Bedrock

Maybe the reason for the stunted progress goes far deeper than we thought. Maybe it is fundamental, going all the way to the scientific bedrock at the true heart of the disease.

—Christofferson, *Tripping Over the Truth*

Come with me now as we board a very special elevator that will take us all the way down to what Christofferson calls "the scientific bedrock that is at the true heart of the disease." Pack a few bags, bring a toothbrush and some spare socks, and prepare yourselves, because it's going to be a long journey down to the guts of the universe. Not to worry—someone has gone to great lengths to furnish us with a high-tech elevator that will take us there. This elevator comes with all the amenities you would want—air conditioning, captain's chairs that convert into beds (like those in first-class sections of airlines), a well-stocked snack bar, TV, internet, you name it. Get in, ladies and gentlemen; sit down, fasten your seat belts, and make yourselves comfortable, as Christofferson closes the doors and presses the button that starts the elevator on it long journey down. Off we go … *whoosh*! Feel those negative Gs!

Fast-forward many hours, and we must be almost there, because the elevator is definitely starting to slow down. Wake everyone up, grab a cup of black coffee, look sharp, and get ready for what's to come. Christofferson presses the button and opens the elevator doors. We hesitate for a moment, then step outside. Wow … what sort of a place is this? There is no light down here, but there doesn't seem to be any darkness either. No colors. No sounds. No textures. It seems all the things that we were used to seeing, hearing, touching, and smelling upstairs have been reduced to their unvarnished scientific ingredients down here. But what exactly are those ingredients? Packets of energy and information? Quantum fluctuations? Dervish dances of elementary particles? A bunch of zeros and ones, like you'd find in the guts of a computer? What's going on down here? Is this some sort of chaos, or is it some sort of order? What? One thing is for sure, however; one thing is for certain: nothing is standing still down here. Everything seems to be in a state of flux, humming and vibrating as it were. The whole place seems to be oriented in the same direction, but what direction?

Who is going to explain this place for us?

Well, for what it's worth, German-born scientist Johannes Dogigli (1915–2002) did explain the bit about the absence of light and color down here. In his book *The Magic of Rays*, Dogigli went to some lengths to point out that "light" and "color" do not exist outside our physiology. What enters the eye consists of invisible wavelengths of electromagnetic radiation. Just packets of energy. Behind the retina, these packets get converted into tiny electric currents that travel along nerve fibers to the centers in the brain, where they first turn into what we would call "light" and "color." Dogigli states:

> Our eye is twice a mirror, a mirror of the soul and a mirror
> of the whole world of rays. Not until things have been
> viewed by our eyes do the processes and phenomena of
> nature acquire the clarity that lifts them out of the world
> of tangible reality into the world of the spirit … Light and
> color are therefore not outside us: we carry them within
> ourselves, for the world around us is blacker than the most
> stygian night.[6]

We seem to be dealing with two versions of the world: an unvarnished version that exists down at the scientific bedrock and a varnished version that exists upstairs where we came from. The former is stripped to the bone. The latter is clothed in flesh. Two versions of the same reality, like

---

[6] Johannes Dogigli, *The Magic of Rays,* Translated from the German and Edited by Charles F. Fullman (New York: Alfred A Knopf, 1961), 33.

the ones featured in *The Matrix* movie, but with one big difference. In *The Matrix*, the cause and effect were purely fictional (there was no connection between the perceived world and those iridescent green emanations). In the real world, the cause and effect *are* factual (there *is* a connection between the perceived world and what's going on at the scientific bedrock). Our human sensations of touch, taste, smell, light, and color may be purely anthropocentric, but they *do* correspond with real phenomena at the cosmic bedrock.

Okay, so there seems to be a connection between what's going on down here and what's going on up there, at least in terms of light and color. But we didn't come all the way down here to talk about light and color! We came here to find the reason for our stunted progress in the war against cancer! So, then, if that reason is hidden somewhere down here, where is it, and what is it? We seem to be on to something, but what? Right now, I'm drawing a blank, and I'm guessing you, dear reader, may be as well. I think we need to call time-out, take a coffee break, and go off on a different tack. We need to simplify. We need to convert the *atomistic* picture that we see down here into a *holistic* picture that our human minds can do business with.

There is this saying, "Can't see the forest for the trees!" I believe this saying applies to our perception of cancer. In our attempt to understand the ontology of the cancer, we can look at one tree at a time, so to speak, or we can look at the forest as a whole. We can take the *atomistic* approach (one tree at a time), or we can take the *holistic* approach (the forest as a whole). The *atomistic* approach would require many years of study in academia, and that's fine and well. The *holistic* approach, on the other hand, could possibly shorten the learning curve. In this publication, we will take the *holistic* approach and make it easier for everyone to apprehend the ontology of cancer.

## Anthropomorphism

*Anthropomorphism* is a compound word made up of two Greek terms, *anthropo* (human) and *morphe* (form). To anthropomorphize is to attribute human form, personality, trait, activity, or other characteristics to nonhuman laws, principles, and forces. We anthropomorphize all the time without knowing it. Gravity causes objects to *fall*, so we talk about "the rise and *fall* of the Roman Empire." We say, "So and so *fell* from grace," or "So and so *fell* in love." Elsewhere, we talk about "Old Man River," "Father Time," or "the devil in the tornado." Statements like these are anthropomorphizations of nonhuman laws, principles, and forces.

The principle that underlies cancer is admittedly a subtle one, at times cryptic and incomprehensible. Not to worry; we will do what great thinkers, writers, poets, philosophers, and prophets have done in their attempts to make the incomprehensible comprehensible. In lieu of the *principle* that underlies cancer, we will posit a *principality* (a principle enforcer). We will give the principle a name, a form, and a personality that our minds can do business with. Granted, scientists tend to take a dim view of anthropomorphisms as such, but to dismiss the approach we are about to take would deprive the human mind of its most potent weapons of insight, introspection, and imagination.

From Greek and Roman personifications of life, death, war, peace, and love as various "gods" to the "cave" in Plato's *Republic*; to John Milton's *Paradise Lost*; to Mary Shelley's *Frankenstein*; to Dante's *Inferno*; to Jules Verne's *From the Earth to the Moon*; to Albert Einstein's *Gedankenexperimente* (thought experiments); to C.S. Lewis's *The Screwtape Letters;* to J.R.R. Tolkien's *Middle Earth*; to H.G. Wells's *The Shape of Things to Come;* to Madeleine L'Engle's *Wrinkle in Time;* to Joseph Campbell's *Power of Myth;* and to George Lucas' *Star Wars,* the classics that have attempted to apprehend the big questions of life have used similitudes, metaphors, analogies, allegories, and anthropomorphisms to draw near to the goal. We will join their ranks by doing the same. As the great Scottish mathematician James Clerk Maxwell once posited his famous "demon" in attempting to apprehend the second law of thermodynamics (Google "Maxwell's demon"), we will now posit an Augustinian "devil" in our attempt to apprehend the ontology of cancer.

## "Cosmic Constable"

Ladies and gentlemen, say hello to the "Cosmic Constable!" The scientific bedrock in which we now find ourselves happens to be his turf, so tread carefully! He is in charge of everything going on down here. In this place, he is all of "big dog," "head honcho," and "shot caller" rolled into one. He is the *archon* (Greek, "ruler") of the rudiments of the perishable universe. But he is no Manichaean devil. He is not capable of bluffing, much less resorting to tricks of craftiness and dissimulation. He is a plain vanilla Augustinian principality (principle enforcer), a blind and amoral executor of the basic laws of physics. Stated figuratively, he is God's "energy czar," hired on by the creator of the universe to maintain the basic order of the universe, the substrate order without which water would run uphill, balls would turn into hedgehogs, and we'd find ourselves in Alice In Wonderland's la-la-land populated by mad hatters, wild queens, ghosts, goblins, boogeymen, and things that go bump in the night—*boo!*

## Authority and Jurisdiction

The Cosmic Constable's authority and jurisdiction is limited to the realms of matter and energy. Those realms have been "given over" to him by the creator of the universe. Okay, so, what's he up to? What is his *modus operandi*? In what way does he go about governing the behavior of matter and energy? More to the point, what's his connection with the way in which cancer misappropriates the free chemical energy in the foods we eat and diverts it into the gaping maws of tumors?

To answer these questions, we have to play detective. We have to don Sherlock Holmes's tweed jacket and deerstalker hat, light his Calabash pipe, grab his magnifying glass, and, accompanied by his trusty friend Watson, set off to investigate the connection between the master sleuth, Cosmic Constable and the disease called cancer.

Watson: "But Sherlock, *is* there a connection?"

Sherlock: "Elementary, my dear Watson, elementary! The cause must precede the effect!"

*Chapter 3*

# The Cosmic Constable

Warburg's approach was guided by the conviction that all processes in living matter obey the laws of physics and chemistry, a view now taken for granted but not generally accepted when he entered the field.

—Hans Krebs, *Otto Warburg*

[T]here is nothing that living things do that cannot be understood from the point of view that they are made of atoms acting according to the laws of physics.

—Richard Feynman,
*The Feynman Lectures on Physics*

To help us understand the ontology of cancer, we have created a *gestalt* and nicknamed it "Cosmic Constable." Here, the term *gestalt* refers to an accelerated method of learning, one that enables the acquisition of the greatest volume of knowledge in the shortest period of time. (Google "definition of *gestalt*.")

Okay, so what can we say about the master sleuth that we have created for ourselves? Who is he, and what's he up to? Let us begin by listing all the things that he is not, starting with the obvious: the Cosmic Constable is not God, much less "the bad side of God." He is not some Gnostic or Manichaean superstition. He is not Zoroaster's *Ahriman;* or Plato's *Demiurge;* or Anaximander's *Apeiron;* or Heraclitus' *Cosmic Fire;* or the Brahmin's *Pradhana;* or the mystic's *World Soul,* or some such construction. Speaking figuratively, and borrowing something from George Lucas's *Star Wars,* we might say that the Cosmic Constable represents "the dark side of

13

the force," being in that sense our "adversary." But he is no Darth Vader. He is not building a Death Star. Stated figuratively, he is God's "energy czar." He can only do what God permits him to do with cosmic energy.

## A Cautionary Note

In everything that we are about to say about the principality that we have just now created, in every way that we are about to describe the activity of the Cosmic Constable, we must always bear in mind that we are dealing with a hyperbole, a fiction, a useful construct, a parable, a metaphor, a caricature—an anthropomorphization of the universe's statistical tendency to disorder (second law of thermodynamics). Obviously, attributing human form and personality to a gestalt such as this does not give life to the fiction, much less invest it with dark purpose or malevolent intent.

There is a place for teleology (purpose and intent), and it's not here. Neither the Cosmic Constable, nor the physical universe, nor the basic laws of physics admit of purpose and/or intent in, of, and by themselves. They are all blind executors of the purpose and intent of God in creating the cosmos, and that's where teleology belongs. The universe doesn't wake up every morning saying, "My purpose is to make general selections in favor of increasing entropy!" The Cosmic Constable doesn't wake up every morning saying, "My purpose is to make statistical selections in favor of more probable states!" Let caution be due here, lest we wonder off into a Manichaean la-la-land and begin investing our Cosmic Constable with devious purpose and diabolical intent.

Okay, so what characteristics might we attribute to something as cold, plain, abstract, amoral, and indifferent as our Cosmic Constable? Well, we might say that he exists on the nonhuman side of the cosmic interface. He lives on the "binary" side of the cosmic computer screen, so to speak. On the human side of the screen, we find the things of the spirit—colors, shapes, forms, ideas, feelings, music, poetry, sports, opinions, beliefs, commentaries, documentaries, videos, movies, and so on and so forth. On the nonhuman side of the cosmic screen, the constable only sees zeros and ones. We are speaking figuratively.

Some science writers have likened the universe to a gigantic computational process in which natural laws function like programs. If the universe were some such super-duper computer, the Cosmic Constable's *modus operandi* would amount to its *default* operating system. In computer jargon, the term *default* stands for a particular setting for a variable that is assigned automatically and remains in effect until overridden. The term *default* can also refer to a rudimentary state to which things will naturally revert in case of higher-level failure. In context, therefore, we could say that the Cosmic Constable's *modus operandi* represents the *modal default* of physical reality, the normative behavior of matter and energy that can only be overridden by the creator of the universe, and that only locally.

## Subtle and Invisible

The Cosmic Constable cannot be seen by the human eye. Scientists may infer his presence by apprehending the laws of physics, and believers may infer his presence by apprehending the Scriptures. Other than that, he remains subtle and invisible. The Cosmic Constable does not think as we do. The expression *cognito ergo sum* ("I think, therefore I am") cannot be applied to the constable, any more than it could be applied to the operating system of a computer. Because we are human, because our inquiry has to be undertaken from a purely anthropocentric point of view, we may refer to the constable as "him" or "he," but we should always bear in mind that we are dealing with an "it."

The dominion of the Cosmic Constable limits itself to that of matter and energy, and the activity of the constable limits itself to that of the stabilization of energy. That's the sum and substance of his *modus operandi: stabilization of energy.* That's his "prime directive," so to speak, his imprimatur.

## Stabilization of Energy

The authority, jurisdiction, and mandate of the Cosmic Constable limits itself to the *stabilization of energy.* He is on the job around the clock, seeing to it that all systems tend toward stabilization. And he is never satisfied with status-quo stabilization. Just because he has reduced some form of energy into a more stable state, it doesn't mean he will take a break. His appetite for energy stabilization is insatiable. He will not be satisfied until he has stabilized all the unstable forms of energy in the universe. He will not rest until he has achieved his ultimate goal of thermodynamic equilibrium. When all the gradients of the universe have been leveled, when all potential differences have been consummated, when the entire aggregate of names and forms have been merged and refunded into undifferentiated stillness, then and only then will the Cosmic Constable be able to retire on his policeman's pension.

## Language of Mathematics

The Cosmic Constable does not speak a human language. His language is the language of pure mathematics. When Galileo opined that the book of nature was written in a mathematical language, he wasn't far from the truth. Neither was Pythagoras when he said, "Number is the measure of all things." Stated figuratively, the "mind" of the Cosmic Constable is the mind of an obsessive, compulsive, left-brained number cruncher. It is the mind of a cyborg-automaton that keeps track of every quantum event in the universe. On his cosmic balance sheet, even the free chemical energy stabilized by the blink of a human eye registers an instantaneous increase in the "stability" (entropy) of the universe. Granted, it's an infinitesimally small increase, but an increase nevertheless.

If the Cosmic Constable were endowed with the gift of human speech (which he is not), his prime directive would be heard echoing throughout the universe:

> Order! Order! Order in the universe!
> Energy must be stabilized!
> Energy must be stabilized.
> Energy must be stabilized!

As the saying goes, "A picture is worth a thousand words," so let us paint a picture of the Cosmic Constable for ourselves. Here he is, the very embodiment of the physics of the universe, clad in traditional attire, helmet with strap under the chin, brass buttons, shiny belt buckle, polished black shoes, whistle, truncheon, stiff upper lip. He is blowing his whistle; swinging his truncheon; directing the cosmic traffic away from initially less probable, lower entropy, less stable energy states toward eventually more probable, higher entropy, more stable energy states. That's how he goes about maintaining the substrate order of the universe. Say hello to the Cosmic Constable, everybody!

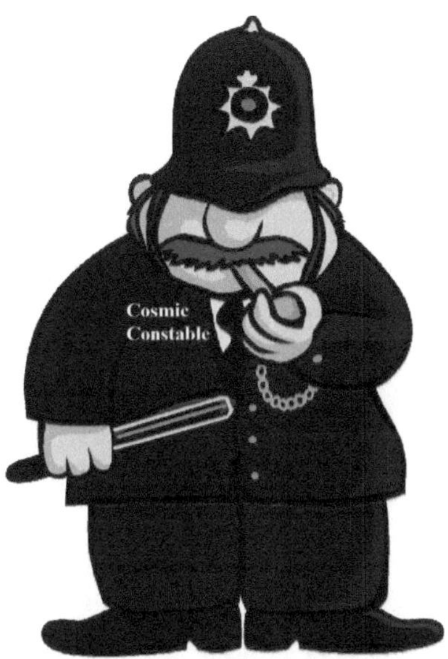


**"Cosmic Constable" = Physics of the Universe**

# Chapter 4

# Order and Disorder

Cancer is a disease of order, and at every step of the way,
it is directed and coordinated from somewhere.
—Travis Christofferson, MS, *Tripping Over the Truth*

What do we mean by "order"? What do we mean by "disorder"? Ever ask yourself? Here's an interesting bit of history. One of Napoleon's army engineers discovered a strange stone near the Egyptian city of Rosetta in 1799. The stone was inscribed with Egyptian hieroglyphics and Greek texts. He had it sent to a museum in France. What later came to be known as the Rosetta Stone had the same narrative inscribed on it in three different languages—two in Egyptian hieroglyphics, which up to that time no one had been able to decipher, and the third in Greek. Because scholars could read the Greek, they could correlate the Greek with the hieroglyphics, and that is how at long last, they were able to decipher the ancient language of Egypt.

In our quest to unravel the riddle of cancer, we seem to have stumbled onto something similar, the same narrative written in two languages, one in the cosmocentric language of the constable, the other in the anthropocentric language of man. The title of the one written in the cosmocentric language of the constable reads *Order*. The title of the other one, written in the anthropocentric language of man, reads *Disorder*. Both are describing the same reality.

## Order or Disorder?

We live in a rational universe created by a rational God; otherwise, science wouldn't have a leg to stand on. Nescience and superstition may posit chaotic principles and arbitrary laws, but within the scientific discipline, the laws that govern the behavior of matter and energy apply uniformly throughout the substrates of space and time. The electron charge on the screen of your cell phone is identical to the electron charge on a quasar on the other side of the cosmos. The proton mass is the same here, there, and everywhere. The speed of light is constant throughout the universe, as is the gravitational constant and a whole lot of other parameters. We don't live in a chaotic universe in which anything goes. We live in a rational universe in which entropy is always increasing, a universe in which things tend to behave predictably.

By now, the behavior of matter and energy is fairly well known to us. We only need to push the envelope a little further to understand the behavior of cancer. This should not be too difficult, given that our bodies are made from the physics of the same universe. Our physiologies are integral components of the behavioral field of the cosmos. Every day, we assimilate free chemical energy in the form of food and eliminate entropy in the forms of heat and waste, yet imagine ourselves to be somehow disconnected from the universe. This is a delusion. There are no disconnects in a rational universe created by a rational God.

## Disorder or Order?

Every day, about 1,600 people die of cancer in the US, and we attribute the phenomenon to some sort of "disorder." This too is delusion. The so-called "disorder" that we might associate with cancer is in reality the substrate "order," without which science and medicine wouldn't have legs to stand on. God himself had to start with the substrate order of dust:

> And the Lord God formed man of the dust of the ground. (Genesis 2:7)

As the Apostle Paul affirms in his letter to the formative church in Corinth:

> There is a natural body, and there is a spiritual body …
> However, the spiritual is not first, but the natural, and
> afterward the spiritual. (1 Corinthians 15: 44–46)

As the Hebrew aphorism also states:

> אִם אֵין קֶמַח, אֵין תּוֹרָה!
> Transliteration: *Im ain kemakh, ain Torah!*
> Translation: "If there is no bread dough (flour), there is
> no Torah!"
> By inference: "The material and spiritual components of
> life are codependent."

## Unraveling the Riddle of Cancer

It is not possible to unravel the riddle of cancer without understanding the substrate "order" that underwrites the phenotype of the disease. Understand the former and you will understand the latter. Understand the "order" that the Cosmic Constable enforces throughout the universe, and you will understand the "mechanism" by which cancer diverts the free chemical energy stored in food into the coffers of fast-growing tumors.

Let's go over what we have covered so far, bearing in mind that we ourselves are unstable forms of energy subject to the "order" that the Cosmic Constable is in business to enforce. What is the prime directive of the Cosmic Constable? His prime directive reads, "Energy must be stabilized!" To remain viable in the universe, the human body must stabilize energy. It must stabilize the relatively unstable free chemical energy stored in food via all its metabolic pathways. If it can do that via its healthy metabolic pathway, it may *in the bargain* be able to remain viable in the universe for the season of a lifetime here on earth. If the healthy metabolic pathway is for some reason impaired, damaged, or blocked, the body can still remain viable in the universe by stabilizing energy via its alternate and more ancient metabolic pathway, "cancer."

You have a puzzled look on your face! You are looking at me and shaking your head. You are saying, "What's this all about? I don't get it! Why would the body do something as silly, stupid, bizarre, and irrational as that?" Let me respond to you in this way: "Because physics trumps biology!"

There is nothing silly, stupid, bizarre, or irrational about a physical system complying with the most basic laws of physics. The body is a physical system. It can only build and maintain biological complexity *in the process of* stabilizing energy. Otherwise, it will fall in disrepair and revert back to the dust of its constitution.

Let's go over that one more time. In order for the physical body to remain viable in a universe such as this, it must stabilize energy for seventy, eighty, ninety, God-willing, a hundred years. If at any point it can no longer stabilize energy via its healthy metabolic pathway, it can at least remain viable in the universe for a shorter period by switching over to its alternate metabolic pathway—cancer. That's the plain logic behind the facts. Otherwise, why would the body bend over backward to build brand-new blood vessels around tumors in order to help them grow faster? Why would the body go to such lengths to prop up a disease that's going to put it six feet under? Answer: "Because it has to!"

So then, cancer is not some diabolical disease transported here by a Manichaean devil hailing from another universe. Although cancer can be initiated by any number of endogenous and/or exogenous causes such as radiation, toxins, asbestos, chemicals, unhealthy foods, smoking, excessive drinking, viral infections, obesity, inflammation, hypoxia, free radicals, and stress, ultimately, the decision to switch to cancer is made by the body itself. Viewed from a purely anthropocentric point of view, the transition from a healthy body to a body riddled with cancer may suggest "disorder." Beneath all appearances, however, cancer is a disease of order. As Christofferson points out:

> Cancer is perceived as a predictable manifestation of a universe that tends toward chaos—one that favors disorder over order ... Although the origin of cancer may be the result of chaos, the disease itself is anything but chaotic. It takes a remarkable amount of coordination to do what

cancer does, to go through the elaborate functionality of the cell cycle flawlessly and repeatedly. To transition to energy creation by fermentation means that the cell must drastically alter its enzymatic profile in an orderly manner. To direct the growth of new blood vessels to feed the growing mass takes an exquisitely complex series of operations. Cancer is a disease of order, and at every step of the way, it is directed and coordinated from somewhere.[7]

Let's see if we can sum it up so far. In order to remain viable for seventy, eighty, ninety, God-willing, a hundred years, the human body must conform to the substrate order of the universe by stabilizing energy. Normally, it can do that via its healthy metabolic pathway. If for some reason or other, the healthy metabolic pathway is impaired, damaged, or blocked, the body can at least remain viable in the universe for a shorter period of time by stabilizing energy via its alternate and more ancient metabolic pathway, the one that we label "cancer." There is nothing new, strange, or complicated about any of this.

---

[7] Travis Christofferson, *Tripping Over the Truth* (White River Junction: Chelsea Green Publishing, 2017), 181.

*Chapter 5*

# Free Energy and Entropy

Entropy is the bioenergetic signature of cancer. Entropy refers to the degree of disorder in systems and is the foundation of the second law of thermodynamics.

—Thomas N. Seyfried,
*Cancer as a Metabolic Disease*

Question: What is *free energy*? Answer: it is the kind of energy that is "available to perform *work*." What *work*? The *work* of building and maintain *structure*. What *structure*? The structure of everything in the universe—galaxies, planets, people, cells. Question: What is *entropy*? Answer: entropy is what gets left behind after free energy gets used up in the performance of *work*. Entropy is the kind of energy that is "no longer available to perform *work*."

> - **Free energy:** Available to perform *work*.
> - **Entropy:** No longer available to perform *work*.

In order for the human body to perform the ongoing *work* of building and maintaining biological complexity, it will need constant infusions of free chemical energy stored in food. The body assimilates free energy, uses some of it to perform the *work* of building and maintaining biological complexity, then stabilizes and dissipates the rest into the cosmos in the form of entropy (heat and waste). This is how the body remains in compliance with the substrate order that the Cosmic Constable enforces. Two things must be noted here:

1) The body can not stabilize (burn off) 100 percent of the free chemical energy stored in food. Why not? Because there would be nothing left to perform useful *work* with.

2) The body cannot utilize 100 percent of the free energy stored in food to perform useful *work* with. Why not? Because the constable's "entropy tax" must always be paid.

## The Body Cannot Be a Simple Heat Engine

Back in 1893, the German-born physicist Adolf Fick pointed out that living cells could not be simple heat engines. What did he mean by that? It might help to look at it in terms of an automobile engine. Yes, the engine does stabilize energy—it produces a lot of heat and waste. Yes, it conforms to the substrate "order" that is being enforced by the Cosmic Constable. But it cannot be just a "heat engine." It must be able to perform *useful work* in the process of stabilizing energy, the kind of *useful work* that enables Mom to drive the kids to school and Dad to drive them to Disneyland.

What is the efficiency of an internal combustion engine? Google it and the answer turns out be somewhere around 50 percent. How much free chemical energy is there in a gallon of gasoline? Google it and the answer turns out to be somewhere around 114,000 BTUs or 120 million Joules (measures of energy). How much of the free energy in a gallon of gasoline does the engine burn off into the cosmos as entropy? 50 percent? How much of that free energy gets left over for mom to drive the kids to school with? 50 percent? Meaning what? Meaning every time mom starts the car, she has to pay the Cosmic Constable a 50 percent entropy tax?

Okay, so Elon Musk comes along with more efficient electric engines. Meaning what? Meaning now we can cheat the Cosmic Constable of his entropy tax? Nope! Not in this universe! We clever humans may find loopholes that enable us to pay the constable his dues at lower tax rates, but in this universe, there is no such thing as a free lunch—100 percent efficient engine. The constable's entropy tax must always be paid.

In principle, the body is just like the automobile engine. It cannot be a simple heat engine—a biological furnace. Yes, it must stabilize energy from cradle to grave. Yes, it produces a lot of heat and waste. But it must also be able to do something besides that. It must be able to perform *useful work* in the process of stabilizing energy, the *useful work* of building and maintaining biological complexity. The body does not produce heat and waste because it is "inefficient." Even the most efficient body in the universe could not convert 100 percent of the free chemical energy stored in food into biological complexity. Why not? Well, again, because the constable's entropy tax must always be paid.

## Entropy Tax

Okay, so what is the entropy tax that the body has to pay the Cosmic Constable in order to remain alive in a universe such as this? What is the tax rate if the body can stabilize, say, one thousand calories of free energy via its healthy metabolic pathway? What is the tax rate if the body ends up having to stabilize the same thousand calories via its alternate metabolic pathway—cancer? Are the tax rates the same? Are they different? What do you think? Any thoughts?

Can a healthy body keep, say, 75 percent of the free energy stored in food for itself before burning the remaining 25 percent off into the cosmos as entropy tax owed the Cosmic Constable? Can the body of a developing embryo keep, say, 80 percent for itself? What about a growing child? A teenager? An adult? Grandma? What about other species—a mouse, a dog, a cat, a horse, an elephant, a shark, a dolphin, a whale? I'm sure you will agree that these are incredibly fascinating questions! In time, it will be up to you millennials to find answers for them. You are venturing out onto undiscovered country, people! You are about to blaze a path that has not been travelled before, leaving a trail that others can follow.

## Theft of Energy by Cancer

From *initiation,* to *progression,* to *invasion,* to *metastasis* and *cachexia,* cancer goes through about five stages. What are the bioenergetic "tax rates" at each stage? What are the numbers? Any ideas? The author has spent hours researching the subject and hasn't been able to find any. The following is pure speculation on my part, offered as an incentive for you millennials to explore the undiscovered country, "to boldly go where no one has gone before!"

**Stage 1 Cancer**

The body gets to keep 50 percent of the free energy stored in food for itself and dissipates the remaining 50 percent into the cosmos as the entropy tax owed the Cosmic Constable. Does this sound right to you?

**Stage 2 Cancer**

The body gets to keep 40 percent of the free energy stored in food for itself and dissipates the remaining 60 percent into the cosmos as the entropy tax owed the Cosmic Constable. Does this sound right to you?

**Stage 3 Cancer**

The body gets to keep 30 percent of the free energy stored in food for itself and dissipates the remaining 70 percent into the cosmos as the entropy tax owed the Cosmic Constable. Does this sound right to you?

**Stage 4 Cancer**

The body gets to keep 20 percent of the free energy stored in food for itself and dissipates the remaining 80 percent into the cosmos as the entropy tax owed the Cosmic Constable. Does this sound right to you? Any thoughts?

**Stage 5 Cancer: Cachexia**

*Cachexia* refers to the severe weight loss that is a characteristic of many debilitating and chronic diseases. It is the dreaded scenario in which the body starves to death for the lack of the free energy it needs to perform the ongoing *work* of building and maintaining biological complexity. With the onset of cachexia, cancer is, for all intents and purposes, terminal. Why? Because the disease is now able to shanghai, steal, divert, stabilize, burn off, and dissipate 90 percent(?) of the free chemical energy stored in food as entropy, leaving very little for the body to survive on. So then when an oncologist says to a cancer patient, "I'm sorry to be the bearer of bad news, but you have six months to live," the oncologist means this: "Your metabolic pathways have been short-circuited by cancer, and the cells of your body are not getting the free energy they need to survive. Your intake of food energy is being diverted into tumors, where it gets processed into heat and waste without doing the *useful work* that is needed to keep you alive. At the present rate of energy depletion, the remaining cells of your body will starve to death within six months."

## Metabolism

The free energy that the body assimilates from food is the kind that is available to perform *useful work*. The used-up energy that the body eliminates in the form of entropy is the kind that is no longer available to perform useful work. The process by which the body assimilates free energy and eliminates entropy is called *metabolism*, from the Greek *metabolē*, which means "change."

The healthy body metabolizes the free chemical energy stored in food via a long and circuitous pathway, using some of it to perform the useful work of building and maintaining biological complexity. The unhealthy body metabolizes the free chemical energy in food via cancer's shorter and more direct pathway, turning more of it into entropy without doing all the *work* of building and maintaining biological complexity. This may be a gross oversimplification, but it describes the principle by which cancer diverts and wastes the free chemical energy stored in food, leaving little for the body to survive on.

## Free Energy Revisited

Free energy is the kind of energy that is available to perform the *work* of building and maintaining structure. As such, it can be said to be the "backbone, support, and scaffolding" of all structure in physical theory. The principle would apply to *all* the structures in the universe, including those of our cells, organs, muscles, bones, members, and brains. Without free energy, there would be no biological structures, no living organisms. For any living thing to remain viable in a universe such as this, it must harvest energy from its environment, break it down (catabolism), reprocess, and reconstitute it (anabolism) into the particular form of free energy that it needs to perform the ongoing *work* of staying alive. (Google "catabolism and anabolism.")

The particular designation of the energy that the body needs to perform the ongoing *work* of staying alive has been given the scientific name of *Adenosine TriPhosphate* (**ATP** for short). Don't let the complicated name throw you. **ATP** is just another designation of energy, and there are many. What do we call the energy that runs our households? We call it "electricity." What do we call the energy that runs our automobiles? We call it "gasoline." What do we call the energy that runs our bodies? We call it *Adenosine TriPhosphate*, **ATP**. (Google the term.)

## Free Energy and Cell Structure

Is there a relationship between **ATP** free energy and cell structure? There would have to be. In fact, you would expect the two to be somewhat fungible, of such constitution that a part or quantity of one could be replaced by a part or quantity of the other. Example: the *structure* of glucose can yield the **ATP** *free energy* that the body can use to build the biological *structure* of the cell. You go from *structure* to *free energy* and back to *structure*. The element of fungibility would look something like this:

Structure ↔ Free Energy ↔ Structure
Chemical Structure → **ATP** → Biological Structure

## Cell Structure and the Cosmic Constable

The principality (principle-enforcer) that we have created for ourselves and nicknamed "Cosmic Constable" is in business to stabilize all forms of free energy in the universe. In principle, we must assume that the element of fungibility is known to him. Stated figuratively, he sees equivalence between free energy and structure. He identifies **ATP** free energy with biological structure, and biological structure with **ATP** free energy. Suffice it to say that he is the great antagonist of both! The two are as thorns in his side. As much as he dislikes free energy, he dislikes structure even more, and the more complex the structure, the greater his dislike. Why? Because there is more work in it for him! Free energy, he can stabilize easily enough, but when it comes to complex structure, he has to break it down into free energy before he can stabilize it into entropy. Mind you, there is nothing personal in any of this. By transforming structure into nonstructure, he is doing his job—stabilizing energy. The fact that we humans would refer to the process as "de-construction" or "de-struction" is beside the point.

The frustration that our friend the Cosmic Constable must feel when he looks at the complex structure of DNA can only be guessed at. The situation can be likened to that of a nefarious jewel thief looking at a priceless diamond on display and wondering how he can overcome the elaborate security arrangements. Suffice it to say that God has found it necessary to place the genetic code under lock and key in an armored safe deep in the nucleus of the cell. The cell may be said to be the sanctuary, the "Fort Knox" of biological life. The healthy cell is like a fenced off area, an "Eden" unto itself, a protected domain that is off limits to the Cosmic Constable. As Israeli physicist Gerald L. Schroeder explains:

> At each step as we go from simple to more complex compounds, we are in a sense swimming upstream in the flow of entropy … [H]ow is it that living organisms regularly produce complex compounds and do so in copious amounts? Life does it by working in the highly protected environment within its cells, by using catalysts that have the ability to select and concentrate the needed chemicals and to increase rates and extents of reactions, and by expending considerable energy to accomplish the tasks. The protected environment needed by life is found within life itself.[8]

In order to remain viable in a universe such as this, life needs a safe and secure castle in which it can use free energy to perform the *useful work* of producing the hundreds of structural and functional proteins needed for orderly diversification and well-regulated growth. Even so, life has to keep an eye out for the constable's shenanigans. The Cosmic Sleuth is always lurking outside, looking for ways to get in. As long as the cell has access to sufficient amounts of **ATP** free energy, it can use it to perform the *useful work* of building and maintaining its fortifications—high walls, watchtowers, and deep moats. But the constable has a few tricks up his sleeve as well. He knows all about the cell's dependence on **ATP** and will not hesitate to employ trebuchets, battering rams, and Trojan Horses to gain entrance into the castle and throw a monkey wrench in the works.

---

[8] Gerald L. Schroeder, *Genesis and the Big Bang* (New York: Bantam Books, 1990), 109.

Let me paint a picture for you. The constable is standing outside the castle wall with bullhorn in hand, issuing his cosmic decree: "Open up! You are unstable forms of energy! I have a cosmic warrant for your arrest!" To which the healthy cell replies, "Go away! I am not violating the first and second laws of thermodynamics!" And so, for the time being, at least, the healthy cell manages to keep the castle gate shut and the meddlesome constable out.

The diseased cell, on the other hand, cannot keep the constable out. The diseased cell does not have access to sufficient amounts of **ATP** free energy to perform the *useful work* of shoring up its fortifications. Somehow, by hook or by crook, the constable manages to wedge a foot in the gate, then a leg, then his whole carcass. Once inside, he flashes a cosmic warrant, seizes the assets, and reprograms the bioenergetics of the cell. What happens next? Well, what happens next runs the whole gamut of what we call "pathology" and "disease."

Perhaps we can apprehend the causes of health and disease in this novel way, everything else being equal. "Health" refers to a condition in which the body has access to the sufficient amounts of **ATP** free energy. "Disease," on the other hand, refers to a condition in which the body does not have access to sufficient amounts of **ATP** free energy. This would seem to suggest that pathology and disease are for the most part caused by impaired **ATP** production.

## The Big Picture

Try to follow the logic of our discourse so far, the logic relating to the principality (principle enforcer) that we have created for ourselves and are calling "Cosmic Constable." Try to see the big picture as he would see it. In looking at the seven billion humans that live on earth, he sees massive concentrations of unstable energy that he must "stabilize." How? Well, in any number of ways. Using diseases like plague and Ebola, for example, he could reduce millions of us to the "stability" of dust overnight. Alternatively, he could use cancer to that end. All he'd have to do would be to sabotage our metabolic pathways, reprogram them to crank out billions of hybrid cells, and bingo, mission accomplished. I see you shaking your head. I hear you say, "But what exactly is the *mechanism* in all this?"

## The Mechanism

Osmosis is the process by which water imperceptibly spreads from the roots of trees to leaves and branches. The term *osmosis* has been used as a metaphor to describe gradual processes by which ideas, knowledge, policies, and trends spread in societies. The metaphor could perhaps be used to describe the *mechanism* by which the substrate order of the universe would gradually and almost imperceptibly bubble up to the surface of human existence in terms of all the pathologies known to man. If osmosis could be used in that sort of context, it could help us to understand the *mechanism* by which the Cosmic Constable gradually and almost imperceptibly nudges the bioenergetics of the human body toward cancer. What do you think? Any thoughts?

With all this in mind, let's see if we can sum up our would-be adversary's mindset and motivation. This is how the Cosmic Constable sees us. This is what he thinks of us. This is what he would be saying to all of us mortals if he were endowed with the gift of speech:

> ➤ Order! Order! Order in the universe!
> ➤ Energy must be stabilized!
> ➤ Free energy must yield to entropy!
> ➤ Instability must yield to stability!
> ➤ Complexity must yield to simplicity!
> ➤ Structure must yield to nonstructure!
> ➤ Differentiation must yield to nondifferentiation!
> ➤ Biology must yield to physics!
> ➤ Organic must yield to nonorganic!
> ➤ Order! Order! Order in the universe!
> ➤ Resistance is futile; you *will* be assimilated!
> ➤ You *will* return to the dust of your constitution!

Of course, this is where the Son of God steps into the breach, confronts the Cosmic Sleuth, and says, "No they won't!" Not to worry, God won't let the constable "assimilate" us. Our Heavenly Father loves us, and He is bigger than the Cosmic Constable. (Romans 8:38–39)

# Chapter 6

# Somatic Mutation Theory of Cancer

The failure to clearly define the origin of cancer is responsible in part for the failure to significantly reduce the death rate from the disease ... How many times must we beat the dead horse before we realize that it will not get up and walk?

—Thomas N. Seyfried,
*Cancer as a Metabolic Disease*

You can't fix something that's broken on the basis of the same set of assumptions that broke it in the first place; you will bounce off the same walls and end up right where you started. You can't start with a flawed theory of cancer, do the same thing over and over again, and expect a different result.

Back in 1987, Dr. Garth Nicolson of the Department of Tumor Biology at the MD Anderson Cancer Center of the University of Texas wrote the following:

The viewpoint that no unitary concept can give a satisfactory explanation of the intimate nature of cancer remains quite valid today.[9]

The failure to clearly define the intimate nature of cancer has been costly. Hundreds of thousands continue to die, and billions of dollars continue to be wasted. Maybe the reason we are losing the war on cancer is because we are

---

[9] G. Nicolson, *Cancer Research* 47 (University of Texas, 1987), 1473–1478.

assuming things that are completely incorrect. To win the war against cancer, we must change some of our most basic assumptions about the disease. As Thomas N. Seyfried states in his magnum opus, *Cancer as Metabolic Disease*:

> I attribute the absence of any real progress in the war on cancer over the last 40 years to the flawed concepts of the somatic mutation theory, and to the failure in recognizing mitochondria dysfunction as a credible scientific explanation for the origin of the disease. This failure is an inexcusable tragedy ultimately responsible for the deaths of millions of cancer patients.[10]

## The Somatic Mutation Theory of Cancer (SMT)

After all the costly research, after all the speeches, after all the pomp and circumstance, after all the backslapping, hype, and hoopla about "breakthroughs," this year another six hundred thousand Americans will probably die of cancer. Something is clearly wrong here. To correct it, we must go through four steps:

1) Begin with a valid premise.
2) Follow through with valid arguments based on the valid premise.
3) Arrive at valid conclusion(s), based on valid arguments, based on the valid premise.
4) Look for evidence that will support our conclusion(s).

The premise must be valid; otherwise, everything that follows—the arguments, explanations, conclusions, pious follies, noble vanities, yada-yada, backslapping, and hoopla—is not going to amount to a hill of beans. Agreed?

---

[10] Thomas N. Seyfried, *Cancer as a Metabolic Disease* (John Whiley & Sons, Hoboken New Jersey, 2012), 204.

## SMT's Assumption

The somatic mutation theory assumes that cancer starts when something goes wrong with genes stored in the nucleus of the cell. That's the basic assumption. But on what premise does the assumption stand? Darwin? Evolution? Natural selection? Genes mutate and get passed along, and you end up with cancer? Is this the assumption that underwrites the somatic mutation theory of cancer? Is this the foundation on which SMT and the entire cancer establishment stands? Let's talk about mutations.

## Mutations

How many DNA copies have there been since the beginning of life on earth? A gazillion-bazillion? Assume that copying errors have cropped up, likely a few bits of information miscopied, or a few bits missing here and there. Assume also that the creative economy of God anticipated these errors and used them as the very basis of what Darwin later stumbled upon and labeled "natural selection."

The copying process involves splitting the DNA strand. An enzyme called *helicase* comes along and performs the *work* of unzipping the strand so that a copy can be made from it. After the copy has been made, an army of DNA-repair proteins go to work to check the fidelity of the copy, and if necessary, they repair errors. Stop and recall, however, that no *work* can be performed without **ATP** free energy. Without **ATP**, the helicase enzyme would not be able to perform the *work* of unzipping the DNA strand. Without **ATP**, the army of DNA-repair proteins would not be able to perform the *work* of checking the fidelity of the copy, much less perform the *work* of correcting errors.

And so, we might suppose that, given the availability of **ATP** free energy, DNA is eminently capable of detecting and repairing miscopied information. Computers do this sort of thing all the time, and they do it with amazing accuracy. Every time you copy something on your computer, laptop, tablet, or smartphone, the operating system checks the fidelity of the copy to make sure it is accurate and tries to fix any errors it may find. If man-made gadgets can perform this sort of *work*, we can reasonably assume that the creative economy of God (aka "evolution") would be able to do the same thing on a much higher order of accuracy and perfection.

The copied and repaired genes could, in fact, be identical to the originals, and they nearly always would be. On rare occasions, however, they would be slightly different, and that slight difference, of course, is the foundation on which Darwin built his Theory of Evolution. Let us put four things into a mixing bowl:

- ➢ Gazillion-bazillion copies of DNA
- ➢ Millions of years
- ➢ Changing environments
- ➢ Competition for limited resources

Mix them all together (mix well!), and let's see what we end up with. Some of the copies would be slightly different. If that slight difference ("mutation") were to confer an advantage to the organism, the trait would be passed along to offspring, and the species would be "selected for survival." Alternatively, if that slight difference were to confer a disadvantage to the organism, *that* would be passed along to offspring, and the species would be "selected for extinction."

Question: Does the somatic mutation theory of cancer have Darwinian legs to stand on? Darwin himself would have been quick to say it does not. Here are his own words:

> Natural Selection acts solely through the preservation of variation in some way *advantageous*, which consequently endure.[11]

> The preservation of *favorable* individual differences and variations, and the destruction of those which are *injurious*, I have called Natural Selection, or the Survival of the Fittest.[12]

---

[11] Charles Darwin, *The Origin of Species* (New York, Modern Library Paperback Edition, 1998), 141, emphasis added.

[12] *Ibid,* 108, emphasis added.

Are the gene mutations that purportedly lead to cancer favorable to the host organism, or are they injurious to the host organism? They are clearly injurious, in which case, evolution would have selected them for extinction long ago! But that's not the case, is it? To provide the somatic mutation theory of cancer with Darwinian legs to stand on, we'd have to assume that diseased cells were being selected for survival and healthy cells were being selected for extinction. What would you call that? Cancer by natural selection? Survival of the fittest, nastiest, most aggressive, most mutated genes?

As Seyfried makes clear in Chapter 15 of *Cancer as a Metabolic Disease,* the devolution of healthy, quiescent, normal cells into rapidly proliferating malignant hybrids would be better explained by the now-debunked theory of Jean-Baptist Lamarck than it would by Darwin's Theory of evolution. So then, just to be clear, just to make sure that we are all on the same page, let us agree that cancer's mutated genes do *not* get selected for survival through a Darwinian mechanism. Meaning what? Meaning there must be a different mechanism involved in their selection.

## SMT on Trial

Let us put the question to the custodians of health, among them the crowned heads of the National Cancer Institute (NCI), the World Health Organization (WHO), the National Institute of Health (NIH), and the Centers for Disease Control (CDC). What exactly is the premise on which the somatic mutation theory of cancer purportedly stands? If it isn't Darwinian evolution, what is it? If cancer is caused by somatic mutations, just how many mutations are we talking about? Exactly which mutation, or group of mutations, can be said to be responsible for the initiation of the disease? Maybe it is for the cancer establishment to stop tripping over the truth and admit that cancer does not start when something goes wrong with the genes that are stored in the nuclei of cells.

SMT fails to make a clear connection between cancer and the ontology of the universe. SMT fails to make a clear connection between cancer and impaired energy production. SMT fails to make a clear connection between cancer and the increase of cellular entropy. SMT stands on feet of clay, and they are crumbling as we speak. The theory cannot deal with and dispose of cancer, because its very premise is flawed. Consequently, the establishment that SMT has fathered has mutated into a billion-dollar, Draconian, tax-consuming bureaucracy "protected by an invisible dome of dogma, large-scale groupthink, and institutional inertia" (Christofferson).

Recall that for 1,500 years, scholars kept making adjustments to Ptolemy's model of the earth-centered universe, until in the end, it collapsed under the weight of its own convolution. Something similar is happening to the somatic mutation theory of cancer today.

# Chapter 7

# Chicken or Egg

In summary, the origin of carcinogenesis resides with the
mitochondria in the cytoplasm, not with the genome in
the nucleus.

—Thomas N. Seyfried

In order for cancer to start, something has to go wrong somewhere, but
what? That's the big question, so let's see if *we* can do a better job of
answering it. To do that, we will have to go through the same four steps:

1) Begin with a valid premise.
2) Follow through with valid arguments based on the valid premise.
3) Arrive at valid conclusions, based on the valid arguments based
   on the valid premise.
4) Look for evidence that will support the conclusion(s).

Let's begin with the premise:

Free energy is the kind of energy that is available to
perform *work*. As such, it can be said to be the "backbone,
scaffolding, and support" of all structure in physical
theory.

Is this premise valid? It would have to be; otherwise, we would be no
better off than the practitioners and purveyors of SMT. Let us start with
the above premise and see where it will lead us. Here we go.

## Argument

Everything we have been talking about here has structure. Cells have structure. DNA has structure. The genome has structure. Structure, structure, structure! Mind-boggling, exquisitely complex structure, the "backbone, scaffolding, and support" of which turns out to be **ATP** free energy. It takes a lot of *work* to maintain the structures of the genes in the nuclei of cells, *work* that cannot be performed without availability of **ATP** free energy. Okay, so where is the **ATP** free energy being produced? Is it being produced in the nuclei of cells? No, it is being produced in the cytoplasm.

Imagine the cell to be an egg. Imagine the nucleus to be the yellow egg yolk. Imagine the cytoplasm to be the egg white. Where is **ATP** being synthesized? In the nucleus (the egg yolk)? No, it is being synthesized in the cytoplasm (the egg white).

Does cancer start when something goes wrong in the nucleus (the egg yolk), or does it start when something goes wrong in the cytoplasm (the egg white)? Does it start with somatic mutations in the nucleus (the egg yolk)? Or does it start with impaired energy production in the cytoplasm (the egg white)? This is the eye-popping, show-stopping, "chicken or egg" question that must be answered if we are to rid the world of the plague of the twentieth century. Seyfried puts the question to those of you who may be a little further along in the sciences:

> If respiratory sufficiency is the origin of cancer, then tumor nuclei should not induce malignancy when placed in cytoplasm containing respiration competent normal mitochondria. Alternatively, if mitochondrial dysfunction is the origin of cancer, normal nuclei should be unable to prevent tumorigenesis when placed into the tumor cytoplasm. I refer to these types of experiments as *nuclear-cytoplasm transfer studies*. What is the evidence from these types of studies that support the metabolic origin of cancer?[13]

---

[13] Thomas N. Seyfried, *Cancer as a Metabolic Disease* (John Whiley & Sons, Hoboken New Jersey, 2012), 160.

Indeed, what is the evidence? Well, the evidence came in the form of two elegant experiments conducted at the University of Vermont and University of Texas. These were two "simple" experiments your author can further simplify by the use of an analogy.

## Egg Yolk and Egg White Analogy

Imagine that we are in a lab working with two eggs. Each egg is a single cell (which is factually true, by the way). The genes are in the nucleus (the egg yolk). The mitochondria that synthesize **ATP** free energy are in the cytoplasm (the egg white). Take a felt-tip pen and mark one egg "healthy" and the other one "malignant."

We will now use a needle to extract yellow yolk from the malignant egg, inject it into the yellow yolk of the healthy egg, and call it *recon*-1. Now we will break *recon*-1, make some scrambled eggs, feed it to lab mice, and see what happens. If cancer is driven by gene mutations in the nucleus (the egg yolk), injecting bad egg yolk into to the good egg yolk should cause the mice to come down with cancer, right? Wrong! Buzzer! No cancer. Happy, healthy mice!

Now extract some egg white from the malignant egg, inject it into the yolk of the healthy egg, and call it *recon*-2. Break *recon*-2, make some scrambled eggs, feed it to lab mice, and see what happens. If cancer is driven by gene mutations in the nucleus (the egg yolk), then injecting bad egg white into the good egg yoke should make no difference, right? Wrong again—buzzer! The mice are now growing tumors!

This was the gist of the elegant experiments conducted at the University of Vermont and University of Texas, with similar results. As Christofferson relates:

> The fact that both groups had demonstrated that the cytoplasm ["egg white"] of a normal cell, with normal mitochondria, could suppress cancer was one thing … But when Schaeffer's [University of Vermont] group proved irrefutably that the cytoplasm ["egg white"] of a tumor cell on its own could initiate and drive cancer, it was impossible to ignore the results … These beautiful

experiments were loaded with theoretical implications, and some would argue that they should have altered the trajectory of a portion of NCI money. But the NCI made the decision that the experiments, even with their astonishing connotations, merited no further exploration. If Seyfried had not dug them up, they may well have been forgotten. Seyfried reflected on the lost importance of the experiments, saying, "In summary, the origin of carcinogenesis resides with the mitochondria in the cytoplasm, not with the genome in the nucleus."[14]

The question one more time: Does cancer start when something goes wrong in the cell's nucleus (egg yolk), or when something goes wrong in the cytoplasm (egg white)? The practitioners and purveyors of SMT maintain that cancer starts when something goes wrong in the nucleus (egg yolk). But hold on a minute! Back up the truck! If free energy is the "backbone, scaffolding, and support of all structure in physical theory," you would expect impaired **ATP** free energy production in the cytoplasm (egg white) to result in impaired genomic structures in the nucleus (egg yolk), wouldn't you? Tom Seyfried explains it in this way (his use of the term *cellular respiration* refers to **ATP** production):

> As DNA repair mechanisms are dependent on the efficiency of respiratory energy production, the continued impairment of respiration will gradually undermine nuclear genome integrity leading to a mutator phenotype and the plethora of somatic mutations identified in tumor cells. Specifically, the integrity of the nuclear genome is dependent on normal cellular respiration.[15]

Can you see the problem with the somatic mutation theory of cancer? If free energy is "the backbone, scaffolding, and support of all structure in

---

[14] Travis Christofferson, *Tripping Over the Truth* (White River Junction, VT, Chelsea Green Publishing, 2017), 146–147.

[15] Thomas N. Seyfried, *Cancer as a Metabolic Disease* (Hoboken, New Jersey, John Wiley and Sons, Inc., 2012), 257.

physical theory," it would follow that the ongoing *work* of maintaining the integrities of structures of the genes in the nucleus (the egg yolk) would depend on the availability of the **ATP** free energy being produced in the cytoplasm (the egg white). Ergo, with any impairment of **ATP** energy production in the cytoplasm, you would expect to find a corresponding impairment of genomic structure (somatic mutation) in the nucleus (egg yolk). Connect the dots, and you may see why cancer cannot be the "gene-driven" disease that purportedly starts in the nuclei of cells. As Seyfried, Christofferson, Know, and many others have repeatedly pointed out, cancer is a *metabolic* disease whose source, origin, and provenance can be traced to impaired **ATP** production in the cytoplasm (egg white).

Let's sum it up in this way: cancer does not begin when something goes wrong in the cell's nucleus (egg yolk). It begins when something goes wrong in the cell's cytoplasm (egg white). Somatic mutations in the nuclei of cells are the *effects* of impaired energy production in the cytoplasm, not the other way around. By fixating on the effects instead of the causes, the practitioners and purveyors of SMT have been putting the cart in front of the horse. That's the reason for our stunted progress in the war against cancer. Tom Seyfried said:

> When will we come to our senses? Until we abandon the idea that cancer is a genetic disease and recognize that mutations are downstream epiphenomena of the disease, there will be little progress in defeating cancer.[16]

---

[16] *Ibid,* 160.

# Chapter 8

# Cancer as Increasing Entropy

A natural process that starts in one equilibrium state and ends in another will go in the direction that causes the combined entropy [disorder] of the system and its environment to increase.

—Halliday and Resnick,
*Fundamentals of Physics*

Don't take the training wheels off yet. To unravel the enigma of cancer, we must fully ground ourselves in the fundamentals of physics. In trying to understand those fundamentals, scientists usually start by breaking them down into two parts: one part they call *system*, and the other they call *environment*. They then try to investigate the way in which the *system* behaves, given the constraints of its *environment*.

For our purposes, the *environment* is the behavioral field of the cosmos (the dominion of what we've been calling "Cosmic Constable"). The *systems* are the cells of our bodies. We are currently investigating the way in which our cells (the *systems*) interact with their environment (the *cosmos*), given the constable's prime directive: "Energy must be stabilized!"

## Entropy in Review

Free energy, we said, is the kind of energy that is available to perform *work*. Okay, so what happens to free energy after it has been used up in the performance of *work*? Does it disappear? Does it get retired to some landfill outside the universe? No, it stays in the universe in the form of entropy. Question: What exactly *is* entropy? Well, again, "entropy is the energy in a closed system that is no longer available to perform *work.*" I see you shaking your head. I hear you say, "We are still talking about cancer, right?" Indeed, we are. Tom Seyfried said:

> Entropy refers to the degree of disorder in systems and is the foundation of the second law of thermodynamics. Szent-Gyorgyi described cancer as a state of increased entropy ...[17]

## Thermodynamics

Just mention the word *heat,* and the first thing that comes to mind is "warmth and temperature." Attention, please: the scientific definition of *heat,* if there be such a definition, has little or nothing to do with "warmth and temperature." In many years of study, your author has yet to come across a rigorous, scientific definition of *heat,* but you may have better luck. (Google "scientific definition of heat.") Galaxies generate *heat* as they process energy. Black holes generate *heat* as they process energy. Stars generate *heat* as they process energy. Engines generate *heat* as they process energy. The human body generates *heat* as it processes energy. Can you think of anything that processes energy and doesn't generate *heat?* But what exactly is *heat?*

Thermodynamics is the branch of science that investigates the relationship between *heat* and other forms of energy. *Thermodynamics* is a compound word made up of the Greek *therme* ("heat") and *dynamis* (energy). And again, please let us not confuse the *thermo* in *thermo*dynamics with "warmth and temperature." The science of thermodynamics assumes several things, among them the following.

> ➢ A sample size of one universe.
> ➢ The universe can be treated as a closed system.
> ➢ The content of the universe can be divided up into two categories of energy: 1, free energy (available to perform *work*), and 2,

---

[17] Thomas N. Seyfried, *Cancer as a Metabolic Disease* (Hoboken, New Jersey, John Wiley and Sons, Inc., 2012), 55.

entropy (already used up in the performance of *work,* hence no longer available).

The first law of thermodynamics states that the overall quantity of energy in the universe (free energy + entropy) remains constant. The second law of thermodynamics states that the quantity of free energy in the universe is *always decreasing.* Why? Well, because it is being used up in the ongoing *work* of maintaining universal structures. As the free energy in the universe gets used up, it gets "stabilized" into entropy, meaning, of course, that the quantity of entropy in the universe is *always increasing.* Call it "the second law of thermodynamics," or call it "increasing entropy." It is what we have been referring to as *stabilization of energy.* Here is what the great physicist Sir Arthur Eddington had to say about it:

> The law that entropy always increases—the second law of thermodynamics—holds I think, the supreme position among the laws of Nature. If someone points out to you that your pet theory of the universe is in disagreement with Maxwell's equations, then so much worse for Maxwell equations. If your theory is found to be contradicted by observation, well these experimentalists do bungle things sometimes. But if your theory is found to be against the second law of Thermodynamics, I can give you no hope; there is nothing for it but to collapse in deepest humiliation.[18]

## All Systems Tend Toward Stabilization

Our friend the Cosmic Constable is on the job 24/7, seeing to it that all universal systems tend toward stabilization. He brings statistical pressure to bear to orient them away from initially less probable, lower entropy, less stable states toward eventually more probable, higher entropy, more stable states, eventually culminating in the most probable, most stable state in the universe: final state of rest, end point of energetic activity

---

[18] Sir Arthur Stanley Edington, *The Nature of the Physical World* (Cambridge University Press, New York, 1928), 74.

beyond which no more change is possible, aka maximum entropy, aka *thermodynamic equilibrium*, aka "death." The Cosmic Constable is on the job 24/7, bringing statistical pressure to bear to encourage physical systems to step down the cosmic energy ladder one step at a time, down, down, down until they reach the last step and then get off the ladder altogether. We are speaking figuratively, of course, and oversimplifying to boot, but the metaphor has basis in reality.

Example: energy in the form of water is "unstable" on a mountaintop. It must stabilize along a gradient common to the whole universe. It must flow down the gradient that leads from initially less probable, lower entropy, less stable states ("mountain heights") to eventually more probable, higher entropy, more stable states ("sea level"). In principle, the Cosmic Constable sees to it that all forms of energy do this sort of thing. That's his job, and he is very good at it. After all, we wouldn't want water to flow uphill, would we? No, we wouldn't. Think of what that would do to our sewer systems! And oh, by the way, because the constable sees to it that water flows from high to low potential, we get to build a "Hoover Dam" that generates the electricity that lights our cities for us. We can do our thing because he does his thing.

You are shaking your head again. I hear you again say, "We are still talking about cancer, right?" Indeed, we are. Energy is energy, irrespective of its outward shapes and forms. The Cosmic Constable doesn't see water flowing down mountainsides or electrons flowing down metabolic pathways. He only sees energy.

## Gradients of the Universe

Water doesn't flow on level ground, and neither do electrons, if you catch my drift. High water on one side of the dam, low water on the other side, and voila, there's the *gradient* that enables energy to flow, generating electricity for us. Cell membranes can function much like dams, providing the needed *gradients* along which energy can travel in our bodies en route to stabilization. High concentration of protons on one side of a membrane, low concentration on the other side, and voila, there's the gradient that enables the free chemical energy stored in food to flow, generating **ATP** for us. As Lee Know explains:

The use of proton pumps to store potential energy in the form of an electrochemical gradient, and then harnessing that energy as it comes across a membrane to create chemical energy, might seem like a strange way to create energy. Yet this seems to be similar across all forms of life on earth.[19]

Allow me to digress for a moment. When Faust asked Mephistopheles (the devil's representative) what he was, Mephistopheles replied, "A part of that force which always seeks evil, and always ends up going good." The energy that we humans have learned to harness is in fact the strength of the principality that we have been calling "Cosmic Constable." In a sense, we have been empowered by our Heavenly Father to harness the constable with bit and bridle and put him to work to plow our fields, turn our engines, light our cities, power the Rolls-Royce, Pratt & Whitney, and General Electric turbines that lift our passenger jets up, up, and away into friendly skies.

We can reliably do our thing, because the constable can be relied upon to do his thing. We have to be careful, however, not to cross the lines that he draws in the sand. The constable is in business to stabilize energy, and he will bring pressure to do just that. If he meets with too much resistance, he may lose his temper, and that can spell no end of trouble for us. All the energy in the universe is at his disposal, and only God stands in the way of what he may or may not do with it. We must tread carefully, wisely, and circumspectly!

We may have learned how to trick the constable into serving our energy needs, but let's not get too cocky or boast about anything, because he has a way of throwing curve balls now and then. I think you know what I mean. In building our power grids, for example, we have to pay a premium in terms of "insulation;" otherwise, he will short circuit the whole thing in no time. The short circuit is, in fact, one of the Cosmic Constable's favorite ploys. He would short circuit (stabilize) every form of energy in the universe along paths of least resistance if he could.

To use cosmic energy, we must construct gradients, resistors, dams,

---

[19] Lee Know, ND, *Mitochondria and the Future of Medicine* (White River Junction, Vermont, Chelsea Green Publishing, 2018), 26.

engines, and machines, and to do that, we must avail ourselves of every ounce of scientific, mechanical, and technological wisdom that our Heavenly Father endows us with. One slip, one error, one oversight, one loose rivet, one flaw in design, and the constable will bring the roof down on our heads. He is just like Murphy, always looking for a weakness to exploit—"Houston, we have a problem!" In principle, he is all of saboteur, thief, terminator, and demolition man rolled into one, always looking for the weakest link in the chain.

## Unrestricted Flow of Energy

The constable desires to see the free and unrestricted flow of energy along a gradient common to the whole universe. He will get upset if the flow gets too restricted somewhere. He will not permit excessive amounts of free energy to accumulate in one place for too long. He will not allow **ATP** free energy to get piled up, bunched up, boxed up, bottled up, dammed up in the human body for too long. No sir! Free energy must *not* be allowed to stagnate for too long. Free energy must be kept moving, flowing down the cosmic gradient that leads away from initially less probable, lower entropy, less stable states to eventually more probable, higher entropy, more stable states.

Granted, there are oodles of free energy bottled up in a single atom, megatons that the constable would like to stabilize in one blinding flash. But he is restrained in that regard. God has placed limits on what he can and cannot do with cosmic energy, and, for the time being at least, the constable is not allowed to stabilize cosmic energy in a series of blinding flashes. (Google "strong nuclear force.") All other forms of energy are fair game, however, including **ATP.**

When we dam up the flow of a river, we are in a sense provoking the constable to his face. When we dam up the flow of energy in our bodies, we are in the same sense provoking him to his face. (Google "obesity and cancer.") Overeating, especially piling on the junk foods, makes it ever so easy for the constable to do his thing with cancer ("garbage in, garbage out"). Mind you, there is nothing personal in what he does. The constable wouldn't know food from fodder, electricity from **ATP!** Energy is energy, and he will bring pressure to bear to stabilize it, regardless of its outward shapes and forms. Certainly, he will not allow its free forms to stagnate in one place for too long. He is constantly looking for opportunities to breach the proverbial dam and restore free flow, so to speak. Don't be surprised to find him attacking the excessive amounts of food energy that we so foolishly divert into our bodies. If he cannot restore free flow through the body's normal metabolic pathways, he will not hesitate to restore free flow via cancer. And we really can't blame him for doing that, can we? No, we can only blame ourselves.

Put yourself in the constable's shoes. If *you* were the Cosmic Constable trying to enforce the most basic order of the universe (no small responsibility!), why would you want to sit around waiting for the free chemical energy in food to be stabilized via the body's long, complicated, circuitous, "healthy" metabolic pathway, if you could get the job done a lot faster via stage-five cancer? Wouldn't make any sense, would it?

*Chapter 9*

# The Probability of Cancer

Just as the constant increase of entropy is the basic law of
the universe, so it is the basic law of life to be ever more
highly structured and to struggle against entropy.
> —Václav Havel

We have all seen turnstiles at bus and railway stations— you know, the one-way gate that lets you in after you insert a coin or a token. The second law of thermodynamics functions much like a cosmic turnstile, a statistical "mechanism" that encourages general movement towards *increasing entropy* (more stable, more probable energy states) while discouraging general movements toward *decreasing entropy* (less stable, less probable energy states). It is important to understand that this "cosmic turnstile" is not merely outside of us. It is internalized in our physiology. Like it or lump it, it is a part and parcel of our entire existence. We are all made from the physics of the same universe, "the dust of the ground" as the Bible puts it (Genesis 2:7), or "the stuff of recycled star dust," as Carl Sagan used to say. The ontology of the cosmos finds expression in our biology and anthropology in subtle ways that we do not yet understand, in subtle ways that we had better start understanding if we are to get past this technological adolescence of ours and rid the world of the plague of the twentieth century.

The principality (principle-enforcer) that we have nicknamed "Cosmic Constable" may be a metaphor, but the associated principle (increasing entropy) has been in effect since the big bang and will continue to be in effect until the universe expires. The fact that the principle is being "enforced" statistically (as opposed to deterministically) makes no difference. The fact that the enforcement thereof cannot be perceived in small samples just means that it is "very subtle" (Genesis 3:1). If it were not so subtle, Plato and Aristotle would have stumbled onto it long ago. But it is subtle—very, very subtle indeed! It can only be apprehended in sufficiently large samples of events, permutations, and iterations.

## Locality and Nonlocality

Look carefully at large samples of both natural and human history, and you may catch a glimpse of the enforcement in question. Five major extinctions. Structure yielding to nonstructure. Complexity yielding to simplicity. The superlative order of life yielding to the diminutive order of dust. Order giving way to disorder; organization giving way to disorganization; culture giving way to barbarism; civilization undergoing to entropic atrophy (pun). "Things fall apart; the center cannot hold" (Yeates); strength wanes away, harmony gives way to disharmony; peace gives way to war; prosperity gives way to poverty; abundance gives way to scarcity; felicity gives way to misery; health gives way to disease. Question: Why do the bad things that we don't want to happen keep happening again and again, and the good things that we want to happen, happen so infrequently? Answer: presumably because the bad things that we don't want to happen embody *more probable states*.

I see you shaking your head again. You are asking the same question: "Are we still talking about cancer?" Indeed, we are. I mean, we are not talking about a chaos of unknown things, are we? No, we are talking about a rational universe created by a rational God. In a rational universe such as this, there are no disconnects between locality and nonlocality, between the anthropology of man and the ontology of the universe. More to your point, there are no disconnects between the biology of cancer and the ontology of the universe.

## Sidebar on Redistributions of Energy

To protect us from the spiritual ramifications of increasing entropy, our Heavenly Father (A) provides us with *special laws* and (B) builds hedges of protection around us. In a purely spiritual context, the *special laws* of God (the Ten Commandments) serve as antidotes to the *general laws* of physics. In as much as the *general laws* of physics would motivate us toward more and more probable (higher and higher entropy) states, the *special laws* of God would motivate us toward less and less probable (lower and lower entropy) states. The statement of principle would go like this: because the *general laws* of physics would orient/drive us toward higher and higher states of disorder, then, therefore, the necessity of the *special laws* of God.

Concomitant to providing us with *special laws* that protect us from the banes of entropy and corruption, our Heavenly Father builds hedges of protection around us, local islands of *decreasing entropy* in a cosmic sea in which entropy is always increasing. But let's have no sloppy science in that regard. Whatever it is that these islands do, they do it with *net conservations of energy and net increases of entropy.* There are no exceptions to the rule. This is a rational universe created by a rational God, an ordered universe in which entropy is always increasing.

Try to picture the cosmos as a great river of change. Locally, there may be small eddies where water molecules rotate upstream. But the river as a whole can only move along a gradient common to the whole universe. What gradient? Well, again, the gradient that leads away from initially less probable, lower entropy, less stable energy states to eventually more probable, higher entropy, more stable energy states. There's no sloppy science in any of this.

## The Creative Economy of God

In the creative economy of God, something local can become more complex at the expense of something nonlocal—*with a net conservation of universal energy and a net increase of universal entropy.* Yes, on this tiny blue planet of ours, evolutionary streams can "flow uphill," so to speak, away from initially more probable, higher entropy, more stable lifeless states toward eventually less probable, lower entropy, less stable living states. This is in part possible because the earth is an open system receiving massive infusions of energy from the sun, infusions that the creative economy of God can redistribute in terms of what Darwin stumbled upon and called "natural selection." But let's have no sloppy science here either. Even as the creative economy of God propels living things "upstream" (like proverbial salmon), it can only do so with *net conservations of universal energy and net increases of universal entropy.* No, my dear religious friend, evolution does not violate the second law of thermodynamics.

## Cancer's Probability

When scientists say "universal entropy is always increasing," they imply that the universe as a whole is moving away from initially less probable unstable energy states toward eventually more and more probable stable energy states. I see you shaking your head again. I hear you say, "Okay, but who sets the standard of probability?" Thank you; this is a very good question! Okay, so who sets the standard of probability? Who determines what is more probable than what? Who is to say if disorder is more probable than order? Who is to say if simplicity is more probable than complexity? Who is to say if repetition is more probable than nonrepetition? Who is to say if proliferation is more probable than quiescence? Who is to say if dust is more probable than DNA? Who is to say if lifelessness is more probable than life? Who can make statements like these without the backing of rock-solid science?

Well, the backing again lies in the proper understanding of *increasing entropy.* Think of it. If there were such a thing as "probability," you would expect it to derive from some sort of background information, some sort of existential default, some larger scheme of things. That background information, that existential default, that larger scheme of things is again *increasing entropy.*

## Background Information

Here is a simple experiment for you millennials. Sprinkle iron filings on a sheet of paper. Gently shake the paper, and observe the patterns. Repeat the cycle many times, and you will note that the patterns are not predictable. They are random, no two the same. That's because there is no "background information" to make them predictable. Now place a magnet under the paper and repeat the experiment. A predictable pattern will emerge every time, communicating something about "background information." The analogy should suffice to demonstrate the relationship between probability and background information.

## Cancer and Background Information

Let's see if we can fine tune the premise of this publication:

> Free energy is the kind of energy that is available to perform the *work* of creating, supporting, and maintaining biological structure.
> Entropy is the kind of energy that is no longer available to perform the *work* of creating, supporting, and maintaining biological structure.
> The probability that universal entropy will increase is 100 percent.
> The 100 percent probability of the nonlocal increase of entropy serves as "background information" for the statistical probability of every local state in the universe, including biological states here on earth.

## Cancer and Quantum Physics

Scientists have always been in the prediction business. Even the Ionian Greeks recognized something similar about universal phenomena and tried to come up with templates that would allow for successful predictions. Not long ago, the template was Newtonian, mainly because scientists were assuming a linear (seamless) continuity between cause and effect. With Max Planck's discovery that microcosmic events involved discontinuous jumps (*quanta*), the Newtonian paradigm was gradually replaced by a probabilistic one. Scientists still recognize the similarity between universal phenomena and have come up with the theory of quantum mechanics (QM) to predict *probable* outcomes, especially at atomic and subatomic levels.

Without delving into the rigors of QM, suffice it to say that a century or so ago, scientists might have said something like this: "Given the linear (seamless) continuity between cause and effect, we predict that such and such will happen with absolute certainty!" Today, they say it a little differently: "Given the quantum discontinuity between initial and eventual states, we predict such and such will happen *with overwhelming probability.*" Probability is the essence of QM.

## Entropy, Probability, and Cancer

In discussing the relationship between thermodynamics and probability, Austrian physicist Ludwig Boltzmann (1844–1906) wrote the following:

> The initial state in most cases is bound to be highly improbable and from it the system will always rapidly approach a more probable state until it finally reaches the most probable state, i.e. that of the heat [thermodynamic] equilibrium. If we apply this to the second basic theorem [second law of thermodynamics] we will be able to identify that quantity which is usually called entropy with the probability of the particular state.[20]

Question: Is there a relationship between entropy, probability, and cancer? If the answer is yes, then perfect health could be the "highly improbable" initial state from which the body would under given circumstances tend to approach "more probable" states of disease until it reached "the most probable state" of thermodynamic equilibrium (aka "death"). But what might trigger the phase transition from the former to the latter?

## Phase Transitions

In a universe in which there is a 100 percent probability that entropy will always increase, you would expect to find local expressions thereof in *phase transitions* from lower to higher probability states. Examples of phase transitions can be found in the natural order. In the flights of starlings, for example, the point at which their initially well-differentiated, individual, complex, random flight patterns suddenly, mysteriously, and magically merge, and they begin to fly as a unit. Looking up at the sky, you could

---

[20] Translation by Kim Sharp and Franz Matschinsky of the 1877 paper of Ludwig Boltzmann, which established the probabilistic basis of entropy. http://crystal.med.upenn.edu/BoltzmannsEntropy3.pdf

easily mistake them for some sort of a moving, twisting cloud. Elsewhere, phase transition can be found in the flashing of fireflies, the threshold beyond which their initially differentiated, individual, complex, random flashes suddenly, mysteriously, and magically synchronize to where they begin to flash in unison. Looking at the mangrove swamp, you'd think the whole place was wired!

Given that atoms, molecules, microorganisms, and metazoans are all made from the physics of the same universe, millennial scientists, anthropologists, and historians will doubtless find many other examples of phase transitions, covering everything from the miniscule to the epic, the mundane to the historical. Consider, for example, phase transitions that trigger viral outbreaks and pandemics; phase transitions that trigger mold, parasites, insect, plant, weed, and pest infestations; and phase transitions that trigger animal stampedes. And it doesn't end there. Given that we ourselves are made from the physics of the same universe, millennial scientists, anthropologists, and historians will no doubt find numerous other examples of phase transitions linking the anthropology of man with the ontology of the universe. Everything from inquisitions that tried to enforce total conformity to stampedes that led to rioting, lootings, burning, and anarchy; to groupthink among capitalists and Marxists; to towing the line in government bureaus; to virtue signaling in media and academia; to panic selling on Wall Street; to craziness "gone viral" in social media.

I see you shaking your head again. You keep asking the same question, "We are still talking about cancer, right?" Indeed, we are. Look carefully at the advanced stages of cancer, and you may see the phase transition from the quiescence of healthy cells to the unbridled proliferation of malignant cells—gone viral. So, then, the take-home message in all this should be clear. Here it is in a nutshell: once large samples of (fill in the blank) go viral, it will be very difficult to stop the phase transition. All the more reason to break up large samples into smaller ones *as soon as possible!* All the more reason to arrest the progress of cancer early in the game, well before the phase transition to metastasis.

## Unbridled Proliferation

In a universe in which there is a 100 percent probability that entropy will always increase, you would expect to find phase transitions from well regulated cell division to unbridled cell proliferation labeled "disease." Beyond a certain point, you would in fact expect unbridled cell proliferation to emerge as a default state. Tom Seyfried puts it this way (read carefully, then read it again):

> A central concept in linking abnormalities of growth signaling and replicative potential to impaired energy metabolism is in recognizing that proliferation, rather than quiescence, is the default state of both microorganisms and metazoans. The default state of the cell is the condition under which cells are found when they are free from any active control. Respiring cells in mature organ systems are largely quiescent because their replicative potential is under negative control through the action of normal mitochondrial function.[21]

Seyfried's reference to "normal mitochondrial function" deserves a great deal of attention here. Given that cells are constituted from the physics of the same universe, keeping their proliferation under tight control is going to take a lot of *work,* the kind of *work* that cannot be done without availability of **ATP** free energy. As long as mitochondria are healthy, they can produce the quantities of **ATP** free energy that cells need to perform the *work* of keeping proliferation under tight control. Question: What happens if mitochondria are damaged, sick, dysfunctional, and can no longer produce sufficient amounts of **ATP** free energy? I will let you answer that question.

---

[21] Thomas N. Seyfried, *Cancer as a Metabolic Disease* (John Whiley & Sons, Hoboken New Jersey, 2012), 208.

# *Chapter 10*

# Stability or Instability?

> If scientists have misunderstood the origin of cancer, then we have lost three decades trying to target mutations that are in fact only a side effect rather than the motor driving the disease.
>
> —Travis Christofferson, MS,
> *Tripping Over the Truth*

What do *we* mean by "stability"? What do we mean by "instability"? Stability is a function of change, isn't it? Or is it? A "stable" system is one that doesn't change much, right? An "unstable" system, on the other hand, is one that's constantly changing. So then, a system that is no longer changing, a system that has reached final equilibrium, a system that is at rest, still, and, for all intents and purposes, dead can be said to be "stable"? Wait just a minute! Back up the truck! Are we now speaking the language of the Cosmic Constable or the language of man? Did we take a wrong turn somewhere?

## The Instability of Life

All things considered, life is an extremely unstable phenomenon in the universe. The season of earthly life that God grants us depends on the maintenance of highly complex, highly structured, highly tensed, highly "unstable" arrangements of material and energetic elements. The magnitude of the complexity of a living cell; the brief and tenuous nature of life; the fine line that separates health from disease; the rapid rate at which flesh will decay after death—all testify to the "instability" of life. This is exactly the sort of "instability" that the Cosmic Constable will try to "stabilize." And I will leave it to you to guess how he will go about doing that.

What do we mean by a "stable" society? Do we mean a society that appears to be "well-ordered" because everyone has the same skin color, looks the same, thinks the same, acts the same, and is a copy of everyone else? No, that's the Cosmic Constable's definition of "stability"! When you and I talk about a stable society, we mean something quite different. We mean complexity. We mean diversity. We mean a fluid, dynamic, noisy, busy, animated, buying, selling, hustling, bustling, moving, shaking, coming-and-going synergy. We mean a *constantly changing* state of affairs that, on the whole, depends on the maintenance of low-entropy, low-probability "unstable" states. This is exactly the sort of "instability" that the Cosmic Constable will try to "stabilize." And I will leave it to you to guess how he will go about doing that.

What do we mean by a "healthy" body? Do we mean a body that appears to be "well-ordered" because all the cells are copies of one another? No, that's a fairly good description of stage-five cancer! When we talk about a healthy body, we mean something quite different. We mean a truly complex, truly extraordinary, truly unconventional, truly uncommon, truly awe-inspiring, truly breathtaking, truly rare and fragile state of affairs in which 37 trillion different cells, two hundred different cell types, and seventy-eight different organs are doing different things in concert. We mean a fluid, dynamic, *constantly changing* synergy that on the whole depends on the maintenance of low-entropy, low-probability, "unstable" states. The word that describes this precariously happy state of affairs is *homeostasis*, from the Greek *homoios* ("same") and *stasis* ("to stand"). This again is exactly the sort of "instability" that the constable will try to "stabilize." And I will again leave it up to you to guess how he will go about doing that.

## Homeostasis

Homeostasis describes the way in which living systems utilize the energy they harvest from their environments to maintain their integrities through myriad regulatory mechanisms. Life does this all the time, utilizing the energy that it harvests from the sun and the food chain to remain viable as long as possible. This is how Tom Seyfried describes it:

> Homeostasis is the tendency of biological systems to maintain relatively stable conditions in their internal environments. Each cell and each organ contributes to the overall homeostasis of the organism.[22]

Obviously, the complex, rare, fragile, tenuous, "unstable" state of biological balance that we call *homeostasis* is not to be confused with what scientists refer to as *thermodynamic equilibrium*. *Homeostasis* describes the process by which the candle of life tries to avoid being blown out by the tempest winds of increasing entropy. *Thermodynamic equilibrium*, on the other hand, describes the end point of energetic activity beyond which no more change is possible. Dead things can be said to be "stable" because they don't change. Living things, on the other hand, can be said to be "unstable" because they are constantly changing (old cells dying and being replaced by new ones). Give the Cosmic Constable a choice between *homeostasis* or *thermodynamic equilibrium*, and which one do you think he will pick?

## Reversal of Conventions

All things considered, it would appear that the conventions of order and disorder are reversed between the Cosmic Constable and ourselves. What the constable would tend to call "order and stability," we would tend to call "disorder and instability," and vice versa. Consequently, we have to be very careful about how we use these terms! The Führer's idea of order and stability had nothing in common with Mother Teresa's. The abomination thought he was bringing order into the world by stamping out the elements of instability. What he actually did was to reduce the continent of Europe to the stability of dust.

I see you shaking your head again. I hear you say: "Okay, this stuff is incredibly fascinating, but what in the world does it have to do with

---

[22] Thomas N. Seyfried, *Cancer as a Metabolic Disease* (Hoboken, New Jersey, John Wiley and Sons, Inc., 2012), 47.

cancer?" Well, again, it has everything to do with cancer. We are not talking about a chaos of unrelated things. The principle that leads to the unbridled proliferation of goose-stepping armies is the same principle that leads to the unbridled proliferation of cancer cells. There is nothing complicated about any of this. In all this, we are looking at the imprimatur of the Cosmic Constable: *increasing entropy.*

## In Summation

Hopefully, we have covered all the things that we need to cover before moving on to mitochondria. Here are the things that we have covered:

- ✓ Energy in general
- ✓ Free energy in particular
- ✓ Entropy in particular
- ✓ Stabilization of energy
- ✓ First law of thermodynamics
- ✓ Second law of thermodynamics
- ✓ Increasing entropy
- ✓ "Heat"
- ✓ Direct relationship between structure and free energy
- ✓ Inverse relationship between structure and entropy
- ✓ Differentiation as a function of low entropy
- ✓ Repetition as a function of high entropy
- ✓ Complexity as a function of low entropy
- ✓ Simplicity as a function of high entropy
- ✓ Redistributions of free energy
- ✓ Evolution as a function of redistributions of free energy
- ✓ Probability in general
- ✓ Probability as a function of "background information"
- ✓ Probability as a function of increasing entropy
- ✓ Quiescence as a function of lower entropy states
- ✓ Proliferation as a function of higher entropy states
- ✓ Order and disorder
- ✓ Stability and instability
- ✓ Homeostasis

Can we now take off the training wheels and start talking about mitochondria? What do you think? I don't know if I've done a good enough job of providing you, dear reader, with the needed framework, but at a certain point, we have to move on, so mitochondria, here we come!

# Chapter 11

# Mitochondria

> Anakin: "Master, sir, I heard Yoda talking about midichlorians. I've been wondering, what are midichlorians?"
>
> Qui-Gon: "Midichlorians are a microscopic life form that resides within all living cells."
>
> Anakin: "They live inside me?"
>
> Qui-Gon: "Inside your cells, yes. And we are symbionts with them."
>
> *Star Wars: Episode I - The Phantom Menace*

Millennials are sometimes referred to as "the *Star Wars* generation." Where did *Star Wars* creator George Lucas come up with the term *midichlorian*? Did he invent it out of whole cloth? No, he didn't invent it out of whole cloth. Mitochondria are submicroscopic organelles that convert the food that animals eat into **ATP** free energy. Plants don't eat food, but they use chloroplast to convert sunlight into the carbohydrates that mitochondria can then synthesize into **ATP**. In a remarkable feat of cinematic insight, Lucas combined the term *mito*chondria with "*chloro*plast" to come up with *midichlorian*. Wonderful! Kudos to Lucas and his team for providing us with the perfect analogy we need to describe the heroic role of mitochondria in this epic saga of ours: *Cancer Wars!*

**Energy is Everything**

Before we start talking about mitochondria, we need once again to remind ourselves about the connection that exists between **ATP** free energy and all living things. Take a look at the abbreviated list below (an unabbreviated version would be hundreds of pages long).

- Cells require **ATP** free energy to remain viable in the universe.
- Cells require **ATP** free energy to divide.
- Cells require **ATP** free energy to ensure copies are accurate.
- Cells require **ATP** free energy to differentiate.
- Cells require **ATP** free energy to *remain* differentiated.
- Cells require **ATP** free energy to control proliferation.
- Cells require **ATP** free energy to maintain genomic stability.
- Cells require **ATP** free energy to build proteins.
- Cells require **ATP** free energy to construct body parts.
- Cells require **ATP** free energy to run their pumps.
- The stomach requires **ATP** free energy to process food.
- The heart requires **ATP** free energy to pump blood.
- The lungs require **ATP** free energy to breathe.
- The muscles require **ATP** free energy to function.
- The pancreas requires **ATP** free energy to synthesize insulin.
- The liver requires **ATP** free energy to detoxify.
- The immune system requires **ATP** free energy to protect the body against germs, pathogens and foreign agents.
- Nerve cells require **ATP** free energy to communicate.
- The eye requires **ATP** free energy to see.
- The ear requires **ATP** free energy to hear.
- The mouth requires **ATP** free energy to speak.
- The hands require **ATP** free energy to touch.
- The legs require free **ATP** energy to walk.
- The lids of your eyes require **ATP** free energy to blink.
- The trillions of cells in your body require **ATP** free energy to make you grow, develop, adapt, and survive.
- The billions of neurons in your brain require **ATP** free energy to process information, to enable you think, to read these words.

Take away **ATP** free energy, and everything on the above list would crumble to dust. From inception to the grave, the cells of our bodies require ongoing infusions of **ATP** free energy, made available to us by our dear and best friends, the midichlorians—beg your pardon, mitochondria. These dear friends of ours have their work cut out for them. Like *Star Wars's* Jedi, they have to do hand-to-hand combat with the constable's stormtroopers. Think of it. Mitochondria are working around the clock to provide us with the useful free energy that we need to survive in a universe such as this, meanwhile Darth Vader, aka Cosmic Constable, is working around the clock to stabilize useful free energy into useless entropy. Needless to say, there is no love lost between mitochondria and the Cosmic Constable. In the epic battle against the dark side of the force, mitochondria are outnumbered and outgunned. And you'd think that we would go out of our way to provide them with the weapons they need to win the war. But no, we ungrateful, stupid, foolish humans go out of our way to poison them with junk foods and toxic chemicals. Shame on us.

## Le Khaim! "To Life!"

In the creative economy of God, mitochondria play a crucial role in enabling us (A) to acquire the gift of life and (B) to use that gift to add value to His creation. When Mom and Dad bring a child into the world, they add immeasurable, inestimable, incalculable value to the Kingdom of God, and this is where mitochondria play a crucial role. At conception, Mom (aka "mitochondrial Eve") donates about one hundred thousand mitochondria to the baby-to-be. Dad only donates about one hundred, most of which don't survive long, and they don't need to. With fertilization complete, Dad's work is done, and Mom's uphill battle begins. Nine months of hard labor against the elemental grain of the cosmos! Nine months of difficult *work* building the most complex array of biological structures in the universe! Not to worry; an army of hard-working, loyal, dedicated, and faithful mitochondria are there to provide Mom with the **ATP** free energy that she needs to perform all that *work* with. Three cheers for mitochondria: hip, hip, hoorah!

The connection between successful pregnancies and the availability of **ATP** free energy can be inferred from what Israeli physicist and Hebrew scholar Dr. Gerald Schroeder has to say about the nine months of gestation:

The brain produces neurons at an astounding rate in the womb. By birth there are one hundred billion. During the nine months of gestation, that averages out to between four and five thousand new nerves each second. Four to five thousand phenomenally complex axon-elongated cells constructed each second, each one racing out to find its target organ. These are guided on their journey by a trillion (a thousand billion!) structural glial cells. Don't just gloss over these fantastically huge numbers. Each cell houses all the complexity we discovered earlier: nucleus, DNA, mRNA, tRNA, ribosomes, motor proteins, ion channels, and on and on. And all are being manufactured at the rate of five thousand per second.[23]

Recall what we said about free energy being the kind of energy that is available to perform *work*. The *work* of building the complex structures Professor Schroeder refers to depends on the *availability* of the pool of **ATP** free energy produced by mitochondria. Free energy, transferred from Mom to embryo, enables the baby's developing brain to perform the difficult *work* of putting together all the complex structures mentioned by Schroeder, such as the nucleus, DNA, mRNA, tRNA, ribosomes, motor proteins, and ion channels. Question: What happens if the pool of **ATP** is less than sufficient?

## The Banes of Poverty and Malnutrition

With the advent of the slave trade in the sixteenth century, most of Europe and the American colonies were imagining that the Black race was genetically inferior to the White race. We have since ascertained that undernourishment of the mother during the nine months of gestation (common among plantation slaves), along with undernourishment of children during their formative years (common in poor regions of the world) can combine to produce physiological and mental deficiencies.

---

[23] Gerald L. Schroeder, PhD, *The Hidden Face of God* (New York: Touchstone, Simon & Schuster, Inc., 2001), 111.

The myth of genetic inferiority went out the window with the advent of modern science.

We are all made from the physics of the same universe (Genesis 2:7), the DNA of the same blood (Acts 17:26–28), species of the same genera—*homo sapiens.* The depravity of man notwithstanding, the Cosmic Constable does not discriminate between our races, cultures, and nationalities. White or Black; Caucasian or Hispanic; European or Asian; Jew or gentile; Israeli or Palestinian; Turk or Armenian; Serb or Croat; Sunni or Shia; Russian or Ukrainian; Indian or Pakistani; Japanese or Chinese; North Korean or South Korean; Hatfield or McCoy, Capulet or Montague makes absolutely no difference to the Cosmic Constable. We are *all* in his crosshairs. He is the blind executor that would reduce *all* of us to the stability of dust. Meaning ultimately, our existential struggle has never been against one another. In the final analysis, our existential struggle has always been against the principality (Cosmic Constable) that discriminates against the "instability" of life. Or as the New Testament puts it:

> For we wrestle not against flesh and blood, but against principalities, against powers, against the rulers of the darkness of this world, against spiritual wickedness in high places. (Ephesians 6:12)

## The Bioenergetics of the Human Body

The 1999 science-fiction movie *The Matrix* depicted a dreadful future in which intelligent machines plugged billions of humans into ghastly biological installations so that their bodies could be used as sources of energy. Estimates are that a healthy body produces somewhere around 1,200 watts of free energy per day, of which about 20 percent (240 watts) gets used by a fully developed brain at rest. A few questions for you millennials: On average, how many of those 1,200 watts get used by a *healthy* heart per day? How many get used by *healthy* lungs per day? How many get used by *healthy* kidneys per day? How many get used by a *healthy* pancreas per day? What are the thresholds that mark the boundaries of health and disease—*measured in units of energy*? Are there significant differences in the bioenergetics of *healthy* and *unhealthy* organs? What about *healthy* and *unhealthy* cells? What about *healthy* and *unhealthy* metabolic pathways? What do the actual numbers look like? Can patterns be inferred from them? When it comes to millennial medicine, sloppy science won't cut the mustard anymore. If cancer is the metabolic disease that you millennials are destined to root out, you will need reliable numbers to work with.

## Cellular Batteries

Let's look at some numbers and make it simple to begin with. The average fully charged AA flashlight battery, for example, can store about four watts of free energy, which would equate with about 12,960 Joules of free energy, which would equate with … how many moles of **ATP**? Let's see you answer the question.

We all know what happens when batteries run down. The flashlight won't work. The cell phone is dead. The car won't start. Well, the trillions of mitochondria swimming around in the cells of our bodies function much like battery chargers. The discharged batteries that they recharge thousands of times every day have been given the scientific name of *Adenosine DiPhosphate* (ADP). Google the term and see what you come up with. Let me help you out here:

- ➢ Mono = one
- ➢ Di = two
- ➢ Tri = three
- ➢ Adenosine TriPhosphate (**ATP**) = "charged battery"
- ➢ Adenosine DiPhosphate (ADP) = "discharged battery"

## Point of Clarification

Attention, please. **ATP** is not free energy in, of, and by itself, any more than a charged battery is free energy in, of, and by itself. Batteries function like containers in which free energy can be stored. **ATP** molecules function like containers in which free energy can be stored. And just as charged batteries can get discharged in the process of performing *work,* or just sitting around, so also **ATP** molecules can get "discharged" in the process of performing *work* or just sitting around. Not to worry; our dear friends the mitochondria are on the job 24/7, recharging ADP back into **ATP**.

Okay, so how do mitochondria recharge ADP back into **ATP**? In principle, they do it the same way that you and I would recharge our cell phones by plugging them into external sources of free energy, such as a wall outlet, generator, power bank, or solar panel. In order to recharge ADP back into **ATP**, mitochondria must likewise "plug into" an external source of free energy, namely the free chemical energy that we ingest in the form of "food." But this, again, is where we let our dear friends down. Instead of providing them with clean sources of food energy to plug into, all too often, we provide them with dirty sources that make them sick. Sick mitochondria cannot provide us with sufficient amounts of the **ATP** free energy that we need to remain alive in a universe such as this. Mitochondria get sick; we get sick. Mitochondria stay healthy; we stay healthy.

## The Dugout and the Playing Field

Borrowing something from the game of baseball, the nucleus of the cell (the egg yolk) has been likened to the dugout in which very little goes on. The cytoplasm of the cell (the egg white), on the other hand, has been likened to the baseball field on which the real action is taking place. The cytoplasm is the place where our dear friends the mitochondria are working around the clock, not only synthesizing **ATP** free energy for us, but regulating cell cycles, monitoring cell division, effectuating millions of interactions between hundreds of proteins, controlling processes by which cells respond to incoming signals, triggering immune responses, initiating apoptosis ... the list goes on and on. Trying to tune in to all that mitochondria are doing in real time would be like trying to tune in to all the crosstalk going on in the radio waves, television waves, shortwave, microwaves, wireless networks, cellular networks, and communication towers in real time. If you and I could do that, we'd go deaf and lose our minds in the process. Well, that's the magnitude of the crosstalk going on in the cells of our bodies every moment of our lives. And our dear friends, the mitochondria, are the ones that have to monitor, regulate, control, and process it. Suffice it to say that we have only scratched the surface of how they go about doing this.

*Chapter 12*

# Bucket Brigade

If all genetic and environmental factors that lead to age-related degenerative diseases converge at the mitochondria, we just need to focus on one organelle.

—Lee Know, ND,<br>*Mitochondria and the Future of Medicine*

In olden days, people would form bucket brigades to put out fires. Mitochondria resort to something similar to convert the food that we eat into **ATP** free energy. The "bucket brigade" that they use is called Electron Transport Chain (ETC for short). What is it, and how does it work?

Let's start on the right foot by bearing in mind that here also we are dealing with the same universal principle, *stabilization of energy*. The Electron Transport Chain's total set of chemical reactions are taking place along a gradient common to the whole universe. What gradient? Well, again, the gradient that leads from initially less probable, lower entropy, less stable energy states toward eventually more probable, higher entropy, more stable energy states.

The relatively unstable free-chemical energy that we ingest in the form of food must be stabilized into entropy if we are to remain viable in a universe such as this. The body can do that via one of two basic metabolic pathways, one "healthy," the other "unhealthy." Either way, the unstable free chemical energy in food *must* be stabilized, or we will run afoul of the Cosmic Constable's prime directive. The metabolic processes by which our bodies utilize cosmic energy involve four basic steps:

1) Food has to be broken down into its energetic components.
2) Those energetic components (principally electrons) have to travel *down* the bucket brigade of the mitochondrial Electron Transport Chain, losing energy along the way.

(Pause and reminder: the law of conservation of energy says energy cannot be lost, only converted into other forms.)

3) The energy that is "lost" along the way has to be converted into protons and pumped into the spaces between mitochondrial membranes. (You will find good illustrations and videos of these online).
4) The pressure of the proton gradient (high concentration of protons on one side of a membrane, low concentrations on the other side) has to be used to drive the ATPase "turbines" that recharge ADP back into **ATP**. (Google *ATPase*.)

## Electron Transport Chain Simplified

The process by which mitochondria reconstitute the free chemical energy in food into **ATP** can be broken down into the four basic steps listed above. All but the first stage takes place within the mitochondrial Electron Transport Chain, and, oh, by the way, it is usually in this initial first stage ("glycolysis") that the energy in food can get diverted into cancer's metabolic pathway. But let's not get too far ahead of ourselves. Let's take it one step at a time, always bearing in mind that it all boils down to the same thing: *stabilization of energy.*

Let's paint a picture that will help us see the simplicity that lies on the other side of all this complexity. Instead of trying to visualize a stream of electrons flowing *down* the gradient of the Electron Transport Chain, let's visualize a stream of water flowing *down* the slope of a mountain, say five thousand feet from peak to sea level. We have high potential at the peak ("unstable energy"). We have low potential at sea level ("stable energy"). According to the Cosmic Constable's prime directive, "Energy must be stabilized!" En route to stabilization, the stream can be diverted into two paths, A or B:

> ➤ A: Useful path to stabilization
> ➤ B: Useless path to stabilization

Path A (analogous to the healthy metabolic pathway) takes the stream through a dozen waterwheels that generate electricity for us. Path B (analogous to cancer's metabolic pathway) diverts the stream over a five thousand-foot sheer cliff, where it plunges useless into the sea. Both pathways stabilize energy. One uses it to generate something useful for us; the other does not. This is the simplicity that lies on the other side of cancer's so-called complexity.

Look at it again. Water flows from high to low potential, losing energy along the way. If the stream gets diverted into path A, the "loss" gets converted into useful electricity by the waterwheels. If it gets diverted into path B, the "loss" gets converted into useless heat-by-friction (tons of water crashing into the sea).

Carry the analogy forward. The free chemical energy in food flows from high to low potential along the gradients of the body's metabolic pathways, losing energy along the way. If it gets diverted into the healthy metabolic pathway, the "loss" gets converted into **ATP** via *oxidation*. If it gets diverted into cancer's unhealthy metabolic pathway, the "loss" gets converted into entropy via *fermentation*. This is a gross oversimplification, to be sure, but it provides us with a fairly good idea of the way in which cancer diverts and wastes the food energy that we all need to remain alive in a universe such as this.

One more time: high potential on the mountaintop, low potential at sea level, and voila, there's the gradient along which energy can flow, generating electricity for us. High potential on one side of the mitochondrial membrane, low potential on the other side, and voila, there's the gradient along which energy can flow, driving the ATPase turbines that enable mitochondria to recharge ADP ("discharged battery") back into **ATP** ("charged battery"). Take a close look at the two metabolic pathways:

> ➤ Path A: Mitochondrial Electron Transport Chain
> ➤ Path B: Cancer

Give the Cosmic Constable a choice between A and B, and which one would he pick?

## A Word or Two about "Efficiency"

We know which metabolic pathway *we* would choose, and we know which metabolic pathway the Cosmic Constable would choose. But can the Cosmic Constable be reasoned with? Well, if he were human, we might be able to reason with him, but he is not human. He is nothing more than a figure of speech that we have created for purposes of our own edification. Suppose, however, just suppose that he were human. How would we go about trying to convince him to choose the healthy metabolic pathway instead of cancer? The dialogue could go something like this:

> Us: "Er … Mister Constable, sir, we know that energy must be stabilized! Yes, yes, of course, energy must be stabilized! Well, the healthy metabolic pathway does stabilize energy, but it makes more efficient use of it!"
>
> Constable: "What do you mean, 'more efficient'?"
>
> Us: "Uh, well, you see, sir, the healthy metabolic pathway can produce a lot more **ATP** in the process of stabilizing energy."
>
> Constable: "So what! I couldn't care less about what you stupid humans consider to be the more 'efficient' ways of stabilizing energy!"

And that's where the conversation would end. It's no use arguing with the principality whose job it is to enforce the most basic order of the universe. All our clever arguments would fall on deaf ears, because the Cosmic Constable couldn't care less about our anthropocentric notions of "efficiency." He does not need to sit around waiting for the free chemical energy in food to traverse the long, complicated, labyrinthine corridors of the healthy metabolic pathway before being stabilized into entropy. From his perspective, the ability of cancer to stabilize energy "efficiently" exceeds that of the healthy metabolic pathway, so that's the pathway he will choose if given the opportunity. And, oh, by the way, all too often it is we ourselves who give him that opportunity.

Another analogy may be sought to help us understand the difference between our anthropocentric notions of "efficiency" and the constable's cosmocentric ones. Let's talk about a gallon of gasoline. Different form of energy, same principle—*energy must be stabilized*. Let us say en route to stabilization, the free chemical energy in gasoline can be diverted into two alternate pathways, A or B:

- ➢ Path A: Automobile engine
- ➢ Path B: Bonfire

The automobile engine has to transfer the gasoline through a complicated system of pumps, fuel lines, fuel injectors, atomizers, and intakes and then mix it with oxygen in the air and precisely time a spark to produce the horsepower that enables Mom to drive the kids to school and Dad to drive them to Disneyland. The bonfire, on the other hand, doesn't have to do any of that. All that the bonfire has to do is to burn the gasoline off as entropy. You already know which pathway the Cosmic Constable would choose, and again, it's no use arguing with him:

> Us: "Er... Mister Constable, sir, we know that energy must be stabilized! Yes, yes, of course, energy must be stabilized! The automobile engine does stabilize energy, but it makes more efficient use of it!"
>
> Constable: "What do you mean, 'more efficient'?"
>
> Us: "Uh, well, you see, sir, the internal combustion engine can produce a lot of horsepower in the process of stabilizing energy, whereas the bonfire cannot!"
>
> Constable: "So what! I couldn't care less about what you stupid humans consider to be the more 'efficient' ways of stabilizing energy!"

You can argue about the "efficiency" of the automobile engine and the "inefficiency" of the bonfire until you are blue in the face, but the constable will light the match every time. You can argue about the "efficiency" of the healthy metabolic pathway and the "inefficiency" of cancer until the cows come home, but the constable will pick cancer every time. By the way, this preference of Cosmic Constable for shorter and more direct pathways of energy stabilization could be said to be the essence of pathology in general—cancer, in particular.

## Olympic Relay Race

There is much more to the Electron Transport Chain than what we have covered here. We have not, for instance, covered the specifics of the way in which electrons get passed *down* the transport chain. Bucket brigade is a good analogy, but it leaves much to be guessed. Perhaps a better analogy would be that of an Olympic relay race, you know, where the first runner hands a baton to the second, the second hands it to the third, and so on and so forth, with the race ending when the final runner crosses the finish line.

Let's change the baton to a hot potato.

At the start of the race, the potato is very hot, and the first runner is anxious to hand it off to the second. By the time the second runner receives the potato, it has lost a little heat, but it's still hot, and he is anxious to hand it off to the third runner. By the time the third runner receives the potato, it's lost a little more heat—and by the time the final runner receives the potato, it has lost most of its heat, and he can comfortably carry it across the finish line.

Figuratively, that is how energy travels *down* the steps of the mitochondrial Electron Transport Chain. The hot potato would correspond with high-energy electrons, and the runners would correspond with the different components of the Electron Transport Chain. But what would the finish line correspond with? Hold on to your hats, because this is where things get a little complicated. The finish line corresponds with one of the most electronegative elements in the periodic table: *oxygen.* Don't panic! Don't change the channel! *Electronegative* just means "a very good receiver of electrons." Oxygen attracts electrons to itself like a magnet. If you ever wondered why iron rusts, or why apples turn brown after they are peeled, it is because the oxygen in air strips electrons out of them, causing them to "oxidize."

## Oxygen

An analogy might be sought to explain the important role played by oxygen in the transport of electrons *down* the bucket brigade of the ETC. Imagine a little boy, Bobby, dropping a dozen ping-pong balls *down* grandma's staircase. Ping, ping, bounce, bounce, *down* they come. Now imagine Bobby collecting them and laying them on level ground. No ping and no bounce! Ping-pong balls don't ping and bounce sitting on level ground; neither do electrons, if you catch my drift. There must be an incline, a gradient, a slope for them to ping and bounce down along. Oxygen provides that incline, as it were. In essence, oxygen "tilts" the ground beneath the Electron Transport Chain so that electrons can "ping and bounce" from high to low potential.

You could say oxygen "collects" electrons in the same way that the sea "collects" streams and rivers. Without sea level, rivers would have no place to flow to. Without oxygen, electrons would have no place to flow to. Without oxygen, unpaired electrons would congregate on level ground, wreaking havoc in terms of free radicals.

Oxygen plays a crucial role in the mitochondrial Electron Transport Chain. If you don't believe that, try holding your breath! Try to understand what Jodi Nunnari, one of the world's leading pioneers in the field of mitochondrial biology at the University of California, Davis, means when she says, "I breathe for mitochondria!" On average, you and I take about sixteen breaths a minute, nine hundred an hour, twenty-three thousand a day, 8.4 million a year. The fact that we have to keep breathing without interruption from cradle to grave gives us a fleeting glimpse of the ongoing *work* that our dear friends the mitochondria have to perform behind the scenes, in order to keep us viable in a universe such as this.

Questions for you millennials: How long does it take for oxygen to travel from your lungs to the mitochondria swimming in the cytoplasm of your cells? Hours? Minutes? Seconds? How long can you survive without oxygen before your body reverts back to the dust of its constitution? Hours? Minutes? Seconds? Let's see you answer these questions.

## Oxidative Phosphorylation

Attention, please—point of clarification: the purpose of the Electron Transport Chain is not to generate **ATP** free energy in, of, and by itself. The purpose of the Electron Transport Chain is to *set the stage* for the generation of **ATP** free energy. An analogy might be sought to clear up any confusion that may exist here. Think of Hoover Dam and the Colorado River. The purpose of the Colorado River is not to generate electricity in, of, and by itself. The purpose of the Colorado River is to *set the stage* for the generation of electricity—to pile up a column of water behind Hoover Dam high enough, at the base of which there will be sufficient pressure to spin the hydroelectric turbines that generate electricity.

Carry the analogy forward. The purpose of the Electron Transport Chain is not to synthesize **ATP** in, of, and by itself. The purpose of the ETC is to pile up a "concentration" of protons behind mitochondrial membranes high enough, at the "base" of which there will be sufficient pressure to spin the ATPase turbines that recharge ADP into **ATP**. We are speaking figuratively, of course, but we should be clear about the coupling mechanisms, nevertheless. Here they are:

> **Hydro-Electric**
> Stage one: Colorado River
> Stage two: Electricity generation
>
> **Oxidative-Phosphorylation**
> Stage one: Electron Transport Chain
> Stage two: Phosphorylation via ATPase

Oxidative Phosphorylation (OxPhos, for short) is an important term that describes the mechanism by which healthy mitochondria go about synthesizing **ATP** free energy for us. (Google *phosphorylation* and *oxidative phosphorylation*.)

## Used-Up Electrons

When electrons have pinged and bounced all the way *down* the Electron Transport Chain, their job is done, and they are no longer needed. Okay, so what are we supposed to do with them? We have to properly dispose of them, right? We can't have gazillions of unpaired electrons running around loose. Unpaired electrons are associated with free radicals. If they are not collected and disposed of properly, they will wreak havoc on everything in sight. Not to worry; as long as oxygen is available, they can be collected and safely disposed of in terms of the carbon dioxide we exhale and the water and waste we eliminate in the bathroom. But what if a heart attack, or a stroke, has rendered oxygen in short supply?

## A Word or Two about Free Radicals

Free radicals are said to be "reactive molecules." What does that mean, "reactive"? Well, it just means "unstable." They are unstable forms of energy, which brings us full circle back to the premise of this publication: *energy must be stabilized*! If energy must be stabilized, and if free radicals are *unstable* forms of energy, our friend the Cosmic Constable would demand that they stabilize themselves. But how would free radicals go about stabilizing themselves?

An analogy might be sought to provide us with a clearer picture here. Think about the wheel of an automobile. Small lead weights positioned around the rim keep it stable as it spins. Say the car hits a bump and one of the weights falls off. The wheel is now out of balance. It is unstable. It starts to wobble. The steering wheel starts to shudder as you get on the freeway. If the wheel were alive, it could stabilize itself by stealing a weight from the wheel of another automobile, which is nonsense, of course. As it turns out, however, unstable molecules ("free radicals") engage in that sort of thing all the time. They steal electrons from nearby molecules in the effort to stabilize themselves. And now, of course, the nearby molecules are unstable, meaning *they* in turn will steal electrons from other molecules, and before you know it, we have cascades of free radicals wreaking havoc on everything in sight. As Winters and Kelley explain:

> A free radical is an atom or compound that is missing one or more electrons and goes about replacing it in an uncontrolled manner. Like a newly single person looking for an instant partner, free radicals are highly unstable and are not selective about where they attain their missing

electron. A free radical will steal an electron from the very first place it can. When free radicals take electrons from proteins, the loss causes tissue stiffening, the disabling of hormones and enzymes, and damage to cell structures …

The cell membrane is one of the most susceptible sites of free radical damage, and once free radicals break down the outer membrane of a cell, they are able to enter and cause damage to the mitochondria inside.[24]

## Free Radicals and Cancer

Do free radicals cause cancer? What do you think? Let's conjure up a worst-case scenario:

➢ Elderly, obese, sedentary
➢ Unhealthy diet, binge eating, sugar addict
➢ Constant stream of electrons entering the bucket brigade with no place to go
➢ No activity, no exercise, not much need for **ATP** free energy, yet more and more unhealthy food ingested
➢ Electron logjam—gazillions of unpaired electrons with no place to go
➢ Cascades of free radicals form, overwhelming and damaging mitochondria.
➢ Mitochondria lose their ability to synthesize **ATP**.
➢ The body can no longer use the healthy metabolic pathway to stabilize energy, but …
➢ Energy must be stabilized!
➢ The body switches over to its alternate metabolic pathway: cancer.

Free radicals could be playing an auxiliary role in tipping the balance in favor of cancer, but there again, so could any number of other things—drugs, smoking, toxic chemicals, asbestos, radiation, and so on and so forth. If cancer were solely caused by free radicals, we'd stand a good chance of rooting it out with antioxidants. What are "antioxidants"? Basically, they

---

[24] Dr. Nasha Winters and Jess Higgins Kelly, MNT, *The Metabolic Approach to Cancer* (White River Junction, Vermont, Chelsea Green Publishing, 2018), 185.

are "electron donors." Imagine mobs of free radicals running around like vandals, looking for electrons to steal. Mr. Antioxidant comes along and says, "Hey, you guys, you don't need to steal electrons from each other. I have lots to spare, and I can donate some to you!" If cancer were caused by free radicals alone, the body's own potent antioxidant (Google *glutathione*), combined with the host of antioxidants available in fruits, vegetables, and over-the-counter supplements, would stand a good chance of rooting it out. But that doesn't seem to be the case, does it? It's not that simple. Cancer is not a simple disease, as Otto Warburg premised decades ago:

> Cancer, above all other diseases, has countless secondary causes. Almost anything can cause cancer. But, even for cancer, there is only one prime cause. Summarized in a few words, the prime cause of cancer is the replacement of the respiration of oxygen in normal body cells by a fermentation of sugar. All normal body cells meet their energy needs by respiration of oxygen, whereas cancer cells meet their energy needs in great part by fermentation … From the standpoint of the physics and chemistry of life this difference between normal and cancer cells is so great that one can scarcely picture a greater difference.[25]

## Summation

Calling it "bucket brigade" or "passing the baton" makes the inner workings of the mitochondrial Electron Transport Chain easier to understand, but the specifics of those inner workings lie beyond the scope of this publication. To explore those specifics, we would have to know everything there is to know about the physical and chemical properties of the compounds involved at a doctorate level. In the broader context of this publication, however, we don't need to know all of that. Suffice it to say that it all boils down to the same thing: *stabilization of energy.*

---

[25] Hans Krebs, *Otto Warburg, Cell Physiologist, Biochemist, and Eccentric* (First published in German in 1979, translated into English and published in 1981, reprinted in 2019 by Ishi Press International, New York and Tokyo, with a new introduction by Sam Sloan), 24.

*Chapter 13*

# Angiogenesis and Metastasis

I would not give a fig for the simplicity on this side of complexity, but I would give my life for the simplicity on the other side of complexity.

—Oliver Wendell Holmes, Jr.

If your author has done a good job of unraveling the enigma of cancer, you, dear reader, should now be in a position to see the simplicity that lies on the other side of its much feared "complexity." Furthermore, you should also be in a position to see the simplicity that lies on the other side of some of its so-called bizarre and inexplicable traits, among them *angiogenesis*, *neovascularization*, and *metastasis*. (Google the terms.) Absent a clear understanding of the bioenergetics of cancer, these traits would indeed seem bizarre and inexplicable, but they are not. The same simplicity lies on the other side of their so-called complexity as well.

Let us again start on the right foot by bearing in mind that we are dealing with the same principle—*stabilization of energy*— and ponder the long, winding, circuitous, intricate, labyrinthine and complicated path that energy would normally have to travel in the body via oxidative phosphorylation. Let us try to understand why the Cosmic Constable would want to avoid as much of it as possible. The following numbers are estimates that you can Google for yourself:

## Average Healthy Human Body

> ➢ About 37 trillion cells
> ➢ Up to several thousand mitochondria in each cell
> ➢ Multiplied trillions of mitochondria in total

Don't just gloss over these huge numbers. Try to see the picture as the Cosmic Constable would see it. The human body *must* stabilize energy in the process of using it. In order to do that, it must "force pump" energy through a lengthy metabolic pathway that leads through trillions of mitochondria, each one offering something by way of resistance, adding up to considerable amount of resistance in total. Imagine trying to pump a hundred gallons of water through a mile-long plastic tube no wider than a drinking straw. Naturally, it would be a lot easier to pump it through a short, wide pipe. The healthy metabolic pathway would be analogous to the mile-long narrow plastic tube. Cancer's metabolic pathway would be analogous to the short, wide pipe. This is a gross oversimplification, to be sure, but it serves to show how cancer can provide the Cosmic Constable with a metabolic path of lower resistance for the stabilization of energy. Cancer takes the shortcut to energy stabilization.

## The Long and Winding Road to Health

In a healthy body, the path that leads to energy stabilization is necessarily long because it must flow through trillions of mitochondria. Healthy cells have to allocate a lot their energy income to the creation and maintenance of biological complexity. Genes have to be turned on and off in precise sequence; lines of code have to be read; rules, regulations, and protocols have to be adhered to; differentiation must be enforced; and uncontrolled proliferation must be restrained, all of which requires a lot of *work*, which in turn requires copious amounts of **ATP** free energy.

In a cancer-ridden body, the path that leads to energy stabilization is shorter. (Otto Warburg said it was "truncated.") Malignant cells have it easy by comparison. They don't have to perform all the difficult and complicated *work* that healthy cells have to perform. All they have to do is to allocate just enough of their energy income to the creation of tumors and burn the rest off in terms of entropy. Cancer bypasses the healthy mitochondrial metabolic pathway and diverts the free chemical energy in food into tumors, where it can be stabilized into entropy more "efficiently." This, too, may be a gross oversimplification, but it does nevertheless serve to explain the difference between our anthropocentric take on cancer and the Cosmic Constable's cosmocentric one. Yes, of course, viewed from our anthropocentric perspective, cancer can be said to be an insidious "disease," and that, it certainly is. Viewed from the constable's perspective, however, cancer is not a "disease." It is the body's alternate and more direct pathway for the stabilization of energy. From the Cosmic Constable's perspective, the human apprehension of cancer as a "disease" is irrelevant and immaterial.

## "Crab"

Cancer is an ancient disease. The fossil record shows it to have been around as long as animals have been around. Centuries ago, the Greek physician Hippocrates (460–370 BC) was baffled by a growth in the breast of one of his patients. The growth was not going away; it was increasing in size. Hippocrates, "the father of medicine," could see that in time, it would encroach on other bodily functions. In examining the growth, he was surprised to discover that the patient's body was supplying it with networks of new blood vessels. The blood vessels were radiating out from the center of the mass, looking like the legs of a crab, so he named it *cancer*, Latin for "crab." That name means nothing to the Cosmic Constable. From his perspective, it is an arbitrary label that we stupid humans have applied to something we don't understand.

## Neovascularization and Angiogenesis

The thing that baffled Hippocrates was, why would the body go to all the trouble of providing a potentially deadly growth with a network of brand-new blood vessels? Twenty-four centuries later, physicians continue to be baffled by the same thing, now referred to as *neovascularization* and *angiogenesis.* Both of these terms describe the creation of brand-new blood vessels around tumors, blood vessels that enable cancer to divert food energy into its own metabolic pathway. Why would the body allow such a thing?

Let us again remind ourselves that the metabolic activity of the human body is not taking place in a vacuum. It is taking place in a universe in which energy must be stabilized. Figuratively speaking, you could explain the bioenergetics of the human body in terms of a circuit plugged into the motherboard of the cosmos. That being the case, all the cells of the body would have to show deference to the "operating system" of the cosmos— meaning they would have to stabilize energy. Naturally, the Cosmic Constable would prefer that they do that along paths of least resistance.

Cancer can provide the constable with the paths of least resistance he prefers, but only if it is supplied with the networks of new blood vessels it needs to divert food energy into its own metabolic pathway. Neovascularization and angiogenesis supply cancer with those blood vessels. There's nothing bizarre or irrational about any of this. This again is the simplicity that lies on the other side of cancer's much misunderstood "complexity."

## Metastasis

From initiation to progression, to invasion, to metastasis, cancer goes through different stages. If caught in time, a tumor with well-defined margins can be surgically removed and the disease stopped in its tracks. But what if the tumor has invaded surrounding tissues? Where are the margins? Where does the tumor end and the healthy tissue begin? Such are the questions that skilled surgeons have to face every day in hospitals around the world. Our hats off to them as they do everything in their power to forestall the phase transition to cancer's deadliest stage: *metastasis*.

Metastasis occurs when a few malignant cells break off from a tumor in one part of the body and spread to other parts. But how is that possible? In order for cancer cells to travel to other parts of the body, they would have to enter and exit ("intravasate" and "extravasate") blood and lymph vessels. This is something that cancer cells cannot ordinarily do. Look at it this way: for you and I to travel around the world, we would need passports issued by the states in which we reside. Likewise, for cancer cells to travel around the body, they would need "passports" issued by the immune system. Ordinarily, the immune system does not issue "passports" to malignant cells. How, then, do cancer cells succeed in spreading throughout the body?

## Macrophage Cells

The group of *myeloid, mesenchymal,* and *stem cells* that do possess "passports" are referred to as *macrophages.* (Google the terms.) What are macrophages? Basically, they are wound-healing cells. The moment you cut your finger, or scrape your knee, or break a wrist, or have a tooth removed, an army of macrophage cells travel to the site to start the healing process (this is a gross oversimplification). Of course, in order to travel to the sites, they would have to enter and exit ("intravasate" and "extravasate") blood and lymph vessels. The immune system provides them with the "passports" they would need for doing that. Figuratively, they show their passports, board the train, travel to the site of the wound, get off the train, show their passports again, and start the healing process.

How can cancer cells travel throughout the body without "passports"? According to one theory, they do it via damaged and/or hybrid macrophage cells. The theory has been around for some time and is explored in greater detail by Tom Seyfried in Chapter 13 of his magnum opus, *Cancer as a Metabolic Disease.* Seyfried mentions the case of a cancer patient who had a tooth removed, and a biopsy from the site of the extraction revealed the presence of cancer cells. Question: How did the cancer cells get there so quickly? In a previous draft of this publication, your author had stated, "by hitching rides on macrophage cells," but the statement was corrected by Professor Seyfried:

> The metastatic cancer cells do not hitch rides on macrophages, as you state. We now know that the metastatic cancer cell arises either from a fusion-hybridization event of a macrophage with a cancer stem cell or directly from a macrophage that's gone rogue due to mitochondrial dysfunction. As the macrophage is already a type of immune cell, immunotherapies will not be effective for the long term management of most

metastatic cancers. Macrophages are powerful suppressors of the immune system.[26]

Think about it. Macrophages would have to be powerful suppressors of the immune system; otherwise, how could they freely travel throughout the body without raising red flags and setting off immune alarms at every turn?

FYI, students more advanced in the science can avail themselves of the latest insights relating to the connection between metastatic cancer cells and macrophages by referring to Figure 3 in a recent open-source paper published by Thomos N. Seyfried (Department of Biology, Boston College) and Christos Chinopoulos (Department of Medical Biochemistry, Budapest, Hungary) at this website: https://www.ncbi.nlm.nih.gov/pmc/articles/PMC8467939/.

## Clever Chameleons

*Chameleon* is a term used to describe the ability of some creatures to blend in with their environment and go undetected by predators. Is cancer able to do something similar? Let's see now; not only are cancer cells able to travel throughout the body without "passports," but upon arrival, they are also able to blend in with different environments and go undetected by the immune system. How is that possible? How could the immune system allow cancer to get away with shenanigans like this?

To answer the question, we would need to once again put on the training wheels and recall what we said about free energy being the kind of energy that is available to perform *work*. In order to prevent cancer cells from getting away with such shenanigans, the immune system would have to perform a lot of *work*, which would require a lot of **ATP** free energy produced by healthy, fully functioning mitochondria. Question: What if mitochondria are sick and not functioning fully? Sum it up in this way:

- ➤ Sick mitochondria = impaired **ATP** production
- ➤ Impaired **ATP** production = impaired immune system
- ➤ Impaired immune system = cancer gets away with shenanigans

---

[26] Personal email, by permission.

## The Stem-Cell Connection

Stem cells function like "generic spare parts" that can be used to rebuild and replace damaged cells. The body stores them in "warehouses" located in bone marrow, skeletal structures, skin tissue, lining of the stomach, liver, and many other places, ready to be recalled and used as needed. Stem cells behave much like chameleons. They are "shape-shifters" in the sense that they can (A) divide and morph into different types of cells and (B) blend in with the different environments without setting off the alarms of the immune system. The reason that macrophage cells can do the same sort of thing is because they are, in part, stem-cell derived. Think of it; they would have to be. How else could they grow new skin cells where you cut your finger, or new connective tissue where you tore a muscle, or new bone and cartilage where you broke your wrist, if they were not stem-cell derived?

Time to play Sherlock Holmes again. Time to don the famous detective's tweed jacket and deerstalker hat, light his calabash pipe, pick up his magnifying glass, and, accompanied by his faithful companion, Watson, ponder the crime scene:

> **Exhibit A:** Macrophage cells are able to able to travel throughout the body and blend in with different environments without being rejected by the immune system.

> **Exhibit B:** Cancer cells are able to travel throughout the body and blend in with different environments without being rejected by the immune system.

> Watson: "I say, old chap, too much of a coincidence, wouldn't you say?"
> Sherlock: "Indeed, Watson; the evidence suggests that cancer cells are able to steal the identities of macrophage cells!"
> Watson: "In that case, what must be done?"
> Sherlock: "Elementary, my dear Watson! We must find ways of preventing the theft as such!"

## The Logic Behind the Facts

One of the most basic mandates of science has always been *to discover the logic behind the facts.* Okay, so what is the logic behind the fact that beyond a certain point the body will sidestep its robust defenses and spread the red carpet before the feet of this devil called "cancer"? What purpose does that serve? Certainly, it serves no *local* purpose. What is the logic behind the fact that beyond a certain point, the body will go out of its way to build brand-new blood vessels around tumors so they can grow faster? What purpose does *that* serve? That serves no *local* purpose either. And what is the logic behind the fact that beyond a certain point, the body will allow malignant cells to spread throughout the body and go undetected by the immune system? Certainly, that serves no *local* purpose either! If these events serve no *local* purpose, we can reasonably assume that they must be serving some *nonlocal* purpose. But what could that be?

If your author has done a good job of peeling away the layers of the onion for you, you, dear reader, should be in a position to answer the question for yourself. If, however, you are still perplexed, still shaking your head, still wanting to know why the human body would want to spread the red carpet before the feet of cancer, I can offer you this simple answer: because everything else being equal, physics trumps biology! Fortunately for us, however, everything else is not equal here. There is God, and His creative economy can override the constable's destructive economy locally. And this is where our Heavenly Father does not force the issue, but rather leaves it up to each of us to choose which economy we would be governed by (Deuteronomy 30:19).

One thing is for sure, however, and one thing is certain: if we choose not to be governed by the creative economy of God, we will—by principle of default—end up being governed by the destructive economy of the Cosmic Constable. Put it this way: if you choose not to be governed by the *special* laws of God, you will be governed by the *general* laws of physics. It's one or the other, with no middle road between the two.

# Chapter 14

# Mitochondrial Munificence

When cells become worn out or damaged beyond repair, they are forced to commit suicide or apoptosis. If the mechanisms regulating apoptosis fail, the one serious consequence is cancer, which is why apoptosis is critical for the integrity and organization of multicellular organisms. This process is controlled by the mitochondria.

—Lee Know, ND,
*Mitochondria and the Future of Medicine*

If the geological column and fossil record are reliable; if God isn't playing tricks with them to confuse atheists, as some young earth creationists suppose, all indications are that the earth is about 4.5 billion years old, and life has been on it for about 3.5 billion years. Remarkably, for its first three billion years, life was single-celled, probably some early form of bacteria. Most people consider bacteria to be the "bad guys," associating them with germs, disease, infections, and so on. All bacteria are not bad guys, however. Some of them are the "good guys" that live in the lining of our stomachs, breaking down raw foods and passing them on to mitochondria. Others are out there doing a marvelous job of cleaning up our oil spills, eating our chemical pollution, processing our factory wastes, treating our nasty sewage—generally helping us clean up the royal mess that we've made of God's green earth.

## Bacteria, Mitochondria, and the Cambrian Explosion

To say that mitochondria are interesting organelles would be an understatement. *Star Trek's* science officer, Mr. Spock, would have referred to them as "fascinating!" Where did mitochondria come from? Some theories suggest that they evolved from early bacteria. Whether they evolved from early bacteria or were a special creation of God is a subject for another book, but one thing is certain: there would have been no Cambrian Explosion without mitochondria. No mitochondria, no Cambrian Explosion, no multicelled organisms, no phyla, no class, no order, no family, no genus, no species—no *homo sapiens.* No mitochondria, no people.

Single-celled organisms are called *prokaryotes.* Multicelled organisms are called *eukaryotes.* (Google the terms.) For three billion years, life on earth was composed of single-celled *prokaryotes.* Then, in the blink of an evolutionary eye, it exploded into all of the mind-bogglingly complex multicelled *eukaryotes* we see in the fossil record. Prokaryotes are relatively simple microscopic life forms that require miniscule amounts of energy to survive (I am using the word *simple* advisedly here because even bacteria contain DNA, and DNA is anything but simple.) Eukaryotes, on the other hand, are orders of magnitude bigger and more complex than prokaryotes, requiring a lot more energy to survive. Think about life's paradigm shift from prokaryotes to eukaryotes, and ask yourself the question: Where did the extra energy come from? Enter mitochondria, as Lee Know explains:

> The acquisition of mitochondria seems to have been *the* decisive moment in the history of life as we know it. If this is true, then the mitochondria deserve all the credit for the abundance of life on Earth as we know it. If not for the mitochondria, the world would not have evolved beyond single-celled bacteria.[27]

---

[27] Lee Know, ND, *Mitochondria and the Future of Medicine* (White River Junction, Vermont, Chelsea Green Publishing, 2018), 10.

## Describing Mitochondria

In attempting to describe mitochondria, one tends to run out of words. To say that they are fascinating, extraordinary, complex, mysterious, generous, humble, altruistic, magnanimous, munificent organelles would be an understatement. The sheer volume of the information that they process would crash our most advanced computers. The length, breadth, height, and depth of the processes that they monitor, regulate, and control boggles the mind. More so, the critical role that they play in directing malignant cells to self-destruct is one of the make-or-break factors in carcinogenesis. (Google *apoptosis*.)

Right now, we really don't know much about these dear friends of ours. We have only scratched the surface of the cytoplasm sea in which they swim. If we were to add everything we know about mitochondria, the sum of our knowledge would amount to the tip of the iceberg, if that. Getting to know these dear friends of ours will no doubt play a great part in shaping the future of medicine. No wonder Lee Know titled his book *Mitochondria and the Future of Medicine.*

## Mitochondrial Mystery

What do we know about mitochondrial division? Do mitochondria divide as a function of cell division (mitosis)? Do they divide independently of cell division? Do they divide pursuant to some sort of a handshake with their host cells? How exactly *do* mitochondria divide? Do they divide by simple fission, like their bacterial ancestors, or through some other mechanism? What controls their rate of division? Is their rate of division in some way triggered by the energy needs of the body? What are the signals that initiate the division? Where do those signals come from? Do mitochondria depend on their host cells for the signaling mechanisms, or do they initiate the signals themselves? The fact that mitochondria cannot be grown in cell-free culture suggests that they do depend on their host cells to some extent, but what is the extent of their dependence? I'm sure you will agree that these are incredibly fascinating questions.

## Mitochondrial Vulnerability

Mitochondria are complex and beautiful organelles, but like all things complex and beautiful, they are especially vulnerable to the Cosmic Constable's assaults. It may come as a surprise, for example, to discover that mitochondria have their own "private" DNA. (Google *mtDNA*.) And this is one of the things that make them so vulnerable to the Cosmic Constable's attacks. We should not confuse the mitochondria's "private" mtDNA with the host cell's "public" nuclear nDNA. Nuclear nDNA is locked away in the cell's nucleus (the "egg yolk") and is generally well protected from the constable's attacks. Mitochondrial mtDNA, on the other hand, is in the cell's cytoplasm (the "egg white"), not so well protected. In order to provide us with the **ATP** free energy that we need to remain alive in a universe such as this, mitochondria have to lower their shields, so to speak, exposing themselves to the constable's "photon torpedoes," as it were.

To understand mitochondrial vulnerability, we must once again put on the training wheels. Free energy, we said, is the kind of energy that is available to perform *work*. In the natural scheme of things, old cells are constantly dying and being replaced by new ones. The replacement procedure (the copying process) involves the *work* of splitting a strand of nuclear DNA, which requires **ATP** free energy. After the copy has been made, an army of DNA-repair proteins have to perform the *work* of checking the fidelity of the copy, which requires **ATP**, and if necessary, perform the *work* of fixing copying errors, which again requires **ATP**. No **ATP**, no *work*, no construction, no repair, no renewal of biological complexity.

## "Catch-22"

How many copies of mtDNA are there in a single mitochondrion? Are these copies all the same? What happens when a cell divides? Do we end up with double the number of mitochondria and double the number of mtDNA? Does an enzyme come along and perform the *work* of unzipping the mitochondrial mtDNA so that a copy can be made? Does an army of mtDNA repair proteins come along and perform the *work* of checking the fidelity of the new mtDNA copies and, if necessary, perform the *work* of repairing errors? Wait just a minute! Back up the truck! Recall that no *work* of any kind can be performed without **ATP** free energy, and mitochondria are themselves the ones that have to synthesize **ATP** in the first place.

Try to see the problem. Mitochondria are the ones that have to synthesize the **ATP** free energy that cells need to perform the *work* of repairing themselves. But who provides mitochondria with the **ATP** free energy that *they* would need to perform the *work* of repairing themselves? What we have here is called a "catch-22." To perform the *work* of repairing themselves, mitochondria would need to produce **ATP** free energy, but the damage they have sustained prevents them from producing **ATP**. (Reminds one of the old saying about a man trying to lift himself up with his own bootstraps.)

## Quiescence vs Proliferation

Uncontrolled proliferation is the well-known characteristic of cancer. What is not so well-known is that mitochondria are the ones that have to keep it under tight control. But at this point we need to stop, call time-out, take a deep breath, and ponder a deeper question. Something big seems to be missing in this discourse of ours, something that we have been taking for granted and glossing over all along. Question: Why would proliferation have to be an issue in the first place? Why would it have to be kept in check?

The answer again lies in the imprimatur of the Cosmic Constable—*increasing entropy.* In a universe in which there is a 100 percent probability that nonlocal entropy will increase, you would expect to find local expressions thereof in terms of uncontrolled proliferation. You would expect to find a "natural" (derivative, default) tendency among organisms to move away from initially less probable *quiescent* states, to eventually more and more probable *proliferative* states. Note what Tom Seyfried has to say about this in *Cancer as a Metabolic Disease.* Read the following carefully, because Seyfried is making a very important observation about the nature of the world, the kind of observation that great thinkers have been known to make:

A central concept in linking abnormalities of growth signaling and replicative potential to impaired energy metabolism is in recognizing that proliferation, rather than quiescence, is the default state of both microorganisms and metazoans. The default state of the cell is the condition under which cells are found when they are free from any active control. Respiring cells in mature organ systems are largely quiescent because their replicative potential is under negative control through the action of normal mitochondrial function.[28]

Seyfried is zeroing in on something that Darwin himself touched on:

In looking at Nature, it is most necessary to keep the foregoing considerations always in mind—never forget that every single organic being may be said to be striving to the utmost to increase in numbers.[29]

## Apoptosis

Apoptosis (pronounced *app'o-toe-sis*) is the process by which mitochondria order malignant cells to self-destruct. Call it "programmed cell death;" call it "programmed cell suicide," *apoptosis* should not be confused with *necrosis*. (Google the terms.) *Necrosis* is what happens when cells are destroyed by things such as trauma, poisons, radiation, or toxic drugs. It is a messy business in which the cell membrane bursts open and spills its toxic content into surrounding tissues. *Apoptosis*, on the other hand, is the well-regulated process by which the cell membrane remains intact as the contents are disposed of and/or recycled in an orderly fashion, and mitochondria are the ones that oversee the process. Mitochondria determine the extent of the damage and, if necessary, initiate the apoptosis cascade. As Lee Know explains:

---

[28] Thomas N. Seyfried, *Cancer as a Metabolic Disease* (John Whiley & Sons, Hoboken New Jersey, 2012), 208.

[29] Charles Darwin, *The Origin of Species* (New York, Modern Library Paperback Edition, 1998), 94.

In apoptosis, the chain of events is perfectly coordinated and leaves no evidence that the cell ever existed. However, there is a price to pay for such a coordinated series of events. All steps along the way require ATP—if the supply of ATP fails to meet the cell's demand, the cell cannot commit apoptosis, and the defective cell is given a chance to run wild.[30]

Lee Know's reference to **ATP** concurs with what we have been saying all along. Free energy, we have been saying, is the kind of energy that is available to perform *work*. As long as healthy mitochondria are producing sufficient amounts of **ATP** free energy, the body can use it to perform the *work* of ridding itself of diseased cells. Question: What if mitochondria have been damaged and can no longer produce sufficient amounts of **ATP**? I will let you answer the question.

## Mitochondrial Munificence

Cancer cells behave like vandals. They replicate like mad, flood the body with "entropy," and eventually bring about the demise of the entire community of cells, including their own. In sharp contrast with the selfish behavior of cancer cells, the behavior of mitochondria is altruistic, even to the point of self-sacrifice. Bear in mind that mitochondria cannot be grown in cell-free culture. Mitochondria cannot survive outside the cell. The cell is their "home sweet home," so to speak. If mitochondria determine the condition of their home to be irredeemable, they will initiate the apoptotic cascade that will bring the roof down on their own heads. Mitochondria will lay down their lives for the benefit of the greater community of cells. (Reminds your author of the words of the dying Spock in one of Gene Roddenberry's *Star Trek* episodes: "The needs of the many outweigh the need of the few.")

---

[30] Lee Know, ND, *Mitochondria and the Future of Medicine* (White River Junction, Vermont, Chelsea Green Publishing, 2018), 120.

## In Summation

However strange, however unlikely, however astounding, however astonishing, however humbling it may seem, at any given moment, trillions of mitochondria are at work in your body, providing you with the **ATP** free energy you would need to think a thought, blink an eye, speak a word, take a step, walk a mile, run a marathon, hit a home run, surf Oahu's Pipeline, climb Everest, play a guitar, compose a symphony, write a novel, start a family, start a business, build a bridge, heal a disease, heal the earth—do all the things that add value to the Kingdom of God. Recalling the words of King David:

> For You formed my inward parts;
> You covered me in my mother's womb.
> I will praise You, for I am fearfully and wonderfully made;
> Marvelous are Your works …
> And that my soul knows very well.
> My frame was not hidden from You,
> When I was made in secret,
> And skillfully wrought in the lowest parts of the earth.
> (Psalm 139:13–15)

Are we beginning to appreciate the critical roles that mitochondria play in our struggle to survive, to remain healthy, to thrive, and to prosper in a universe such as this? As Seyfried keeps reminding us, "energy is everything," and mitochondria are the organelles that provide us with it in the form of **ATP**. Should we not return the favor by providing them with the healthy sustenance they need in order to be able to do all that they do for us?

*Chapter 15*

# Millennial Science of Complexity

Number is the measure of all things.
— Pythagoras

The author may be accused of simplifying too much; anthropomorphizing too much; colloquializing too much; digressing too much; wandering off topic at times; getting too folksy at times; using too many hyperboles; using too many analogies; and so on and so forth (guilty as charged), but the one sin that he does not want to be accused of is peddling sloppy science to millennials. We can't afford to be sloppy in the way in which we make the connection between free energy, mitochondria, and human health. Recalling the words of Pythagoras, "Number is the measure of all things," we need to make that connection in terms of real numbers, but right now, we can't do that, because science has yet to come up with workable ways of defining and measuring *complexity*. Granted, we can use our God-given faculties of sight, sense, smell, taste, and common sense to make intuitive judgments about what's healthy to eat and what isn't, but as of yet, we can't link our intuition to the millennial science of *complexity*. As of yet, the science does not exist.

## Building Blocks of Complexity

What do you need to build a house that can withstand the ravages of time? You need timber, brick, mortar, concrete and steel. You can build your house out of mud and it may stand for a while, but when the storm comes, it will crumble. What do you need to build strong cells that can withstand the ravages of disease? You need proteins, carbohydrates, amino acids, lipids, vitamins, minerals, trace elements, micronutrients, and myriad other building blocks. You can build your cells using junk foods, but when cancer comes, it will put you six feet under. You can't fortify your body by eating junk foods. You need complex ingredients to do that.

Consider, for example, the important roles played by trace elements like chromium, cobalt, copper, fluorine, iodine, iron, manganese, molybdenum, selenium, and vanadium. Some have been described as "the spark plugs of life." Others are known to act as catalysts, speeding up chemical reactions that would otherwise require weeks to complete. Magnesium, for example, plays an important role in assisting mitochondria to produce **ATP**. Zinc plays an important role in synthesizing proteins, facilitating nutrient absorption, and regulating many other processes.

When it comes to the pattern of complexity we call "health," every component of the body has to work in orchestration with every other component. The operative word here is *orchestration*. Think about the London Symphony Orchestra performing Beethoven's Ninth. You have a musical score. You have a conductor. You have finely tuned musical instruments. They all have to work together to produce a magnificent symphony. The same goes with health. The musical score is DNA. The precisely tuned instruments are the cells. The musicians are the mitochondria. They all have to work together to produce the *complexity* that we label "health." Unfortunately, science has yet to explain what we mean by "complexity," let alone come up with ways of defining and measuring it.

## Two Apples

Imagine that we are in a lab working with two different apples. Which one would be "healthier"? Well, that would depend on any number of things, wouldn't it? If we had a millennial complexity protocol to work with, we could measure the complexity of each apple, find out which of the two had a higher complexity value, and judge it be more conducive to health. Unfortunately, we can't do that right now, because science is lagging behind in that respect. Time to push the envelope.

## Millennial Homework Assignment

It is time to push the envelope of science toward clearer understandings of the causes of disease in general—cancer, in particular. To do that, you millennials will have to come up with workable ways of defining and measuring complexity. They don't have to be perfect; they just have to be workable. It's a difficult task to be sure, but doable, nevertheless. I say doable because at this point, we can posit an inverse relationship between entropy and complexity. If entropy can be measured in terms of numbers, so can complexity. With this in mind, let us review the thesis of this publication and see where it will lead us. Here we go:

> ➢ **Free energy** is the kind of energy that is available to perform the *work* of building and maintaining biological complexity. It is therefore plausible to posit a direct relationship between free energy and complexity in biological systems, everything else being equal.
> ➢ **"Complexity,"** underlined three times in red ink and not to be confused with "complication," may be defined in terms of the *quality* and *specificity* of information in biological systems, where high *quality* and high *specificity* would correspond with high levels of complexity, and low *quality* and low *specificity* would correspond with low levels of complexity, everything else being equal.
> ➢ **The quality and specificity of information** in biological systems may be measured in terms of … (fill in the blank as a part of your millennial homework assignment).

This all sounds complicated. It *would* be complicated if the universe were a chaos of unknown things, but it is not. We live in a *rational* universe created by a *rational* God; otherwise, science wouldn't have a leg to stand on. Look at the word *rational* for a moment. *Rational* can take on different meanings; it can mean "reasonable," for example, or "sensible," i.e., "So and so is a rational person." In science, however, the word takes on a different meaning, as with "rational numbers." Given the rationality of the universe in which we find ourselves, we should be able to express complexity in terms of real numbers.

## Redundancy

In many respects, redundancy can be said to be the inverse of complexity. An analogy might be sought to show what we mean by "redundancy." Imagine that we are standing in front of two walls of equal mass: a relatively simple wall made of bricks and a relatively complex wall made of stone. The brick wall was built in a single day and contains a lot of redundancy (repetition). The stone wall, on the other hand, the kind that you may see around estates of millionaires, was built by a skilled mason, took three months to create, and contains a lot less redundancy (no two stones are exactly alike). Both walls contain the elements of complexity, among them:

- ➤ Numbers relating to constitution of structure
- ➤ Numbers relating to redundancy of structure
- ➤ Numbers relating to the quantities of free energy used to perform the *work* of creating their structures

The attendant hypothesis might read something like this:

- ➤ Structures with low redundancy would tend to have higher complexity values than structures with high redundancy, everything else being equal.

## Measures of Complexity

We use various units to measure things with. We use meters to measure length, liters to measure liquids, volts to measure electricity, Celsius to measure temperature, Joules to measure energy, and Newtons to measure force. To come up with ways of measuring complexity, we will need a unit of measure. Since no such unit exists presently, let me make one up for you: "Avigdor" (Avi, for short.)

I don't know what the Avi numbers will look like fifty years from now, but I'm guessing that (A) they will have many decimal points, and (B) they will all fall short of the positive integer of 1. Of course, the reason they will fall short of the positive integer of 1 is because in this universe, there can be no such thing as permanent complexity. Look at it this way: You can't keep all the money you earn, you have to part with some of it in terms of taxes. So too with complexity. You have to part with some of in terms of the entropy tax owed the Cosmic Constable. Consequently, nothing in the universe will be found to have a complexity value of Avigdor 1.0000000. Everything in the universe will be found to have a complexity value short of Avi 1.0000000.

## Back to our Two Apples Analogy

Let us apply the hypothesis to our two apples illustration. It is conceivable that fifty years from now, the millennial science of complexity will be able to make routine assessments that might go something like this (I'm making up the scenario and the numbers and fantasizing to boot):

> Scientists at the *Institute of Planetary Complexity* in Jerusalem, Israel, measured the complexity values of the two apples in question with the following results. They found 0.0070000 Avigdors of complexity in sample A and 0.0065000 Avigdors of complexity in sample B. These values would suggest that mitochondria would prefer the former to the latter, everything else being equal.

Naturally, all complexity values would have to be accompanied by time stamps, hence the need for many decimal points. The apple that has a complexity value of 0.0070000 Avigdors at this point in time may have a complexity value of 0.0069999 Avigdors an hour from now, the 0.0000001 loss of complexity attributable to entropy tax paid to the constable as a function of time.

## Millennial Complexity Protocol

In chemistry, a *mole* is the unit used to measure the amount of substance in samples of matter. For the time being, and until a better unit can be devised, we can use the *mole* as a measure of the amount of substance in foods as well. Let's start pushing the envelope by asking a series of rhetorical questions. Here we go.

How many Avigdors of complexity are there in a mole of refined white flour? How many Avigdors of complexity are there in a mole of refined white sugar? Some profound intuition would seem to be telling us that these values would tend to be very low, but right now, we can't back up our intuition with real numbers.

How many Avigdors of complexity are there in a mole of GMO (genetically modified) corn? How many Avigdors of complexity are there in a mole of non-GMO corn? Is there a difference between the two complexity values? If so, what would be the extent of the difference, and how would it affect mitochondrial function? Again, some profound intuition would seem to be telling us that mitochondria would prefer non-GMO to GMO, but right now, we can't back up our intuition with real numbers.

How many Avigdors of complexity are there in a mole of GMO soybeans? How many Avigdors of complexity are there in a mole of non-GMO soybeans? Is there difference between the two complexity values? If so, what would be the extent of the difference, and how would it affect the ability of mitochondria to synthesize **ATP** free energy? Put it this way: How would it affect the health and well-being of millions around the world?

Here are a few more examples; try to come up with your own. How many Avigdors of complexity are there in, say, a mole of organically grown and processed California Nonpareil almonds, when no pesticides or chemicals are used? How many Avigdors of complexity are there in a mole of nonorganic California Nonpareil almonds, grown using pesticides and chemicals? Is there a difference between the two complexity values? Again, some intuition would seem to be telling us that organic almonds would be blessed with higher complexity values than nonorganic, but right now, we can't back up our intuition with real numbers.

How many Avigdors of complexity are there in a mole of commercially hydrogenated salad oil? How many Avigdors of complexity are there in a mole of cold-pressed virgin olive oil? Is there a difference between the two complexity values? If so, what would be the extent of the difference, and how would that difference affect mitochondrial function?

How many Avigdors of complexity are there in a mole of hamburger taken from commercially caged cattle loaded with steroids, hormones, and antibiotics? How many Avigdors of complexity are there in a mole of hamburger taken from grass-fed, free-range cattle? Is there a difference between the two complexity values? If so, what would be the extent of the difference, and how would it affect mitochondrial function? Put it this way: How would it affect the health and well-being of the millions who daily frequent McDonald's restaurants around the world?

How many Avigdors of complexity are there in a mole of commercially farmed salmon? How many Avigdors of complexity are there in a mole of Alaskan wild salmon? Is there a difference between the two complexity values? If so, what would be the extent of the difference, and how would the difference affect mitochondrial function?

What about the complexity values of other food products? What about seeds? We don't know. What about vegetables? We don't know. What about fruit? We don't know. What about bread? We don't know. What about eggs? We don't know. What about dairy? We don't know. What about poultry? We don't know. We don't know; we don't know; we don't know! And the penalty we pay for not knowing, we pay in terms of pathology, disease, and cancer.

## Feed the Children

Questions for you millennials: Are toddlers around the world being fed infant formulas containing GMO corn and soy ingredients? How are these formulas going to affect their long-term health and well-being? Any thoughts? A few decades ago, the synthetic estrogen drug *diethylstilberstrol* (DES for short) was approved by the United States Food and Drug Administration for use in the livestock industry to make cattle put on weight faster. In one of the greatest blunders in the history of science and medicine, between 1938 and 1971, DES was also administered to pregnant women to enhance growth in the womb and prevent miscarriage. The mistake resulted in widespread birth defects and a veritable epidemic of infantile cancers. (Google *DES babies*.)

## Feed the People

Since the 1950s, the FDA has continued to approve the use chemical formulations for use by the livestock industry, some of which can make cattle put on weight a lot faster. Among them are *estradiol, progesterone, testosterone, zeranol, androgen trenbolone acetate,* and *progestin melengestrol acetate.* Question: Do these formulations interfere with the ability of mitochondria to synthesize **ATP** free energy in the bodies of the humans who consume the meat? Put it this way: Is there linkage between the FDA's continued approval of such chemicals and the increased rates of diabetes, heart disease, and cancer? What do you think? The European Union apparently thinks so. In 1989, the EU banned the importation of American beef laden with such chemicals. The reason for the ban was in part due to scientific research commissioned by the EU finding sufficient evidence to consider the hormone drug *estradiol* to be "an outright carcinogen." No kidding, an outright carcinogen! You can find a summary of the finding at this website:

https://www.ncbi.nlm.nih.gov/pmc/articles/PMC1115840/.

If you are wondering why the FDA would allow the use of such drugs, just follow the money trail. Follow the bread crumbs all the way from the boardrooms of food and beverage giants to the offices of lobbyists on K-Street in Washington, DC, to the hallowed halls of the United States Congress right next door, and from there, to the cancer wards in which balding patients are injected with chemo poisons and afterwards handed buckets to throw up in. This is the price that we pay for living in the dark ages of science and medicine. Shame on us.

## A Word or Two about Complexity and Information

In discussing complexity and information, we should be clear about a couple of things. For starters, we should be clear about the deeper meaning of the word *information.* This is a compound word made up of the prefix *in,* followed by the noun *formation,* which most dictionaries define as "the structure or arrangement of something." When scientists of the caliber of Richard Feynman and Norbert Weiner talk about "information," they have in mind something other than the superficial meaning of the word.

Another thing we should be careful about is to avoid confusing *quantity* of information with *quality* of information. The operating system of your old desktop PC used a relatively high *quantity* of relatively low-*quality* information (so-called "spaghetti code"). In order to process all the redundant information, your old desktop had to perform a lot of *work*, which required a lot of energy, which meant you had to plug it into a wall. The operating system of your latest smartphone, on the other hand, contains a relatively low *quantity* of relatively high-*quality* information (much less redundancy). Your latest iPhone doesn't have to perform all the unnecessary *work* that your old desktop had to perform; consequently, it requires a lot less energy to perform the work with, even though in terms of processing information, it can outperform your old desktop by orders of magnitude. So then, if we were to infer a relationship between complexity and information, our inference would have to relate to the *quality* rather than the *quantity* of information.

It has been said that the human body is the most efficient processor of energy in the universe. If this is true, then I will leave it up to you to infer the relationship between **ATP** free energy, complexity, and health. Certainly, you would expect **ATP**-rich healthy cells to have much higher complexity values than malignant cells.

## In Summation

It takes a lot of *work* to build and maintain the level of complexity we call "health," and none of that *work* can be performed without the availability of the free energy that healthy mitochondria synthesize for us in the form of **ATP**. Let's connect the dots:

> ➤ Healthy mitochondria = healthy people
> ➤ Sick mitochondria = sick people

## Chapter 16

# Critical Path to Rooting Out Cancer in Twenty-Five Years

With malice toward none; with charity for all; with firmness in the right, as God gives us to see the right, let us strive on to finish the work we are in.

—Abraham Lincoln

### Millennial Challenge

Root out cancer within twenty-five years. Divide those twenty-five years into incremental steps with clear goals, benchmarks, and deadlines.

### Required Reading

Be it in schools, academia, or elsewhere, when it comes to the acquisition of knowledge, certain publications fall under the category of "required reading." The pre-mitochondrial struggle against cancer has been covered by hundreds of books, most of which fail to take the journey down to the scientific bedrock of energy. The post-mitochondrial struggle has been covered by a relatively short list of books that should be considered "required reading" by all who would aspire to live in a cancer-free world. Among them should be:

*Tripping Over the Truth*
*How the Metabolic Theory of Cancer is Overturning One of*
*Medicine's Most Entrenched Paradigms*

Travis Christofferson, MS
Published in 2017 by Chelsea Green Publishing

*Mitochondria and the Future of Medicine*
*The Key to Understanding Disease, Chronic Illness, Aging,*
*and Life Itself*
Lee Know, ND
Published in 2018 by Chelsea Green Publishing

*Cancer as a Metabolic Disease*
*On the Origin, Management, and Prevention of Cancer*
Thomas N. Seyfried, PhD
Published in 2012 by John Wiley and Sons, Inc.

## Prospectus

- **Sick planet:** Studies indicate that in the near future half of all men and a third of all women in the US will develop some form of cancer in their lifetime. (Google it.) Numbers don't lie, and they are getting to be alarming. Without a sea change in our understanding and treatment of cancer, all the families of the earth stand to be affected by the disease.

- **The economic cost:** Since President Nixon's "War on Cancer" in 1971, the federal government has doled out well over one hundred billion taxpayer dollars for cancer research, with little to show for it in terms of annual deaths. The cost of some cancer drug treatments can exceed $100,000 a year. (Google "the cost of cancer.") All indications are that things will get worse before they get better. Without a sea change in our understanding and treatment of cancer, the disease will drive people into bankruptcy, place unsustainable burdens on economies, and tear apart the fabric of human societies.

- **The human cost:** Present day "slash, burn, and poison" strategies of dealing with cancer are often accompanied by horrendous side effects that reduce patients to empty shells of their former selves. Without a sea change in our understanding and treatment of cancer, the disease will bring with it hopelessness, despair, ruin, and desolation on unprecedented scales. More so, it will weigh down the conscience of the whole human race, spelling the failure of our species to overcome a scourge bent on our destruction.

## Winning the War

### Ideal Outcomes

- **Reversing the trends:** Imagine a world in which cancer rates are plummeting. Imagine!
- **Reducing the cost:** Imagine a world in which billions of dollars used for cancer research and treatment can now be put to better use in optimizing human health and well-being. Imagine!
- **Restoring human dignity:** Imagine a world in which the cancer wards have been emptied! No more fear, no more doubt, no more dread associated with the word *cancer*. No more pain, no more chemo poisons, no more radiation, no more surgery, no more tearful parents watching their balding children stagger about in hospital gowns with terrified looks on their faces. Imagine the revival of hope! Imagine the restoration of confidence in the ability of the human race to overcome and dispose of the plague of the twentieth century. Imagine!

### Seven Obstacles

1: Nescience
2: Flawed theory
3: Flawed research
4: Vested interests
    i: Food and beverage
    ii: Pharmacological
    iii: Chemical
5: Uninformed public
6: Money, finances, revenue
7: Loss of momentum

## Obstacle #1: Nescience

*Nescience* has been variously defined as "nonscience," "deficit of knowledge," "false consciousness," or "ignorance." Whereas science tries to pursue truths that liberate and set free, nescience pursues falsehoods that bind and oppress. Nescience builds pedestals of human arrogance that science tears down. There have been many such pedestals, and thankfully, most of them have been torn down by science. One such pedestal had us believing that we were the center of the universe—torn down by science. Another had us believing that evolution had granted us privileged status on the tree of life—torn down by science. A few have yet to be torn down, chief among them the one that would have us believe that we enjoy some sort of arbitrary privilege and exemption in the universe. This is a delusion based on nescience.

The privileges, exemptions, and liberties that we *do* enjoy as men and women created in the image of God are neither arbitrary nor gratuitous. They are *spiritually* derived and can only be found within the sanctuary of the Kingdom of God. Outside that sanctuary, we are so many pounds of unstable energy earmarked for "stabilization."

Your author would define nescience as a lack of knowledge, an unawareness or an outright ignorance of the relationship in which we image bearers of God stand to a cosmos in which entropy ("disorder") is always increasing. The idea that we can live in a universe such as this and yet enjoy arbitrary privilege and exemption is arrogant assumption based on nescience. This is one of the last pedestals of arrogance that science needs to tear down, and the sooner the better.

Science itself tells us we are made from the physics of a rational universe in which everything is connected together, a universe in which even the blink of a human eye results in a net conservation of universal energy and a net increase of universal entropy. In a rational universe such as this, there are no ultimate schisms, no ultimate rifts, no ultimate fractures, no ultimate derangements, no ultimate disconnects between anthropology of man and the ontology of the universe—the bioenergetics of cancer and the basic laws of physics.

Let us take a look at the way in which nescience goes about trying to deal with cancer. Writ large in the fabric of the universe are words that describe its ontology: *Energy must be stabilized!* In order to remain viable in a universe such as this, the human body must stabilize energy. If it cannot stabilize energy via its normal metabolic pathway, it can at least stabilize it via cancer. Let's go over that one more time. In order for the physical system of the human body to remain viable in a universe such as this, it must be able to stabilize energy. If it can stabilize it via its healthy metabolic pathway, it may be able to remain viable for seventy, eighty, ninety—God willing, a hundred years. If it cannot stabilize energy via its healthy metabolic pathway, it can at least stabilize it via cancer and continue to remain viable, albeit for a far shorter period of time.

Against a background such as this, the practitioners of SMT (somatic mutation theory) come along and try to kill cancer by surgery, chemotherapy, and radiation. Against the same background, the practitioners of MMT (mitochondrial metabolic theory) come along and try to kill cancer by starving it of its fermentative fuels (glucose and glutamine). You don't need to be Einstein to see that neither approach is tenable.

One more time: in order to remain viable in the universe, the body *must* stabilize energy! If it fails to do that via one metabolic pathway, it can do it via another metabolic pathway. If it fails to stabilize energy via either of its metabolic pathways something worse than cancer will come along and put it six feet under. Let me put it to you this way: if the body fails to stabilize energy via any of its metabolic pathways, a red flag will alert our friend the Cosmic Constable, and he will restore the noncompliant physiology to the dust of its constitution. Dust to dust, ashes to ashes. And the hospital's certificate will list the cause of death as ... what? "Complications due to cancer"?

Stop! Hold on! Back up the truck! What are we saying? Are we saying cancer should not be treated, because if all else fails, the body can use it to remain viable in the universe for a little while longer? Negative! That is *not* what we are saying! What we are saying is this (read carefully): by all means, attack cancer with everything you've got. By all means, try to kill cancer via the existing standard of care. By all means, try to kill cancer by starving it of its fermentable fuels. Do it, not as the be-all and end-all of the Hippocratic Oath, but as the first step in *repairing the healthy metabolic pathway so that the body would not need to switch to cancer in its effort to remain viable in the universe!*

As to which is the more effective standard of care, I can only offer you this opinion: when science replaces nescience, it will replace the ineffective standards of care with effective ones. That is the length, breadth, height, and depth of what your author has to say about "standards of care." When in doubt, consult your physician. Check.

## Obstacle #2: Flawed Theory

Probably the next big obstacle standing in the way of rooting out cancer relates to flawed theories of the disease. The somatic mutation theory (SMT) that has been driving billion-dollar cancer research now appears to be flawed. As Travis Christofferson documents in *Tripping Over the Truth*, despite all the costly research undertaken to validate SMT, to date, neither a single mutation nor any combinations of mutations have been clearly shown to be at the root of the initiation of the disease:

> No researcher today can point to any single mutation or any combination of mutations and say with confidence that it alone is the cause of cancer. Nor can researchers point to a series of cellular systems rendered dysfunctional by mutations and make the same claim with confidence.[31]

Increasingly, indications are that cancer is a *metabolic* disease, meaning it relates to the way in which the body utilizes ("metabolizes") the free chemical energy in foods to maintain its physiological homeostasis without running afoul of the most basic laws of the universe. This being the case, understanding the way in which the body utilizes energy requires a thorough review of the concept of energy in general, free energy in particular, as well as the critical role played by mitochondria in reconstituting the free chemical energy in food into **ATP**—subjects we have hopefully done a good job of covering in previous sections of this book. Check.

---

[31] Travis Christofferson, *Tripping Over the Truth* (White River Junction, VT, Chelsea Green Publishing, 2017), 181.

## How to Replace SMT with a Metabolic Theory

Replacing SMT with a mitochondrial metabolic theory (MMT) won't be easy. Human nature being what it is, the problem can be summed up in the word *inertia*, loosely defined as "a general tendency for things to remain unchanged." The practitioners and purveyors of SMT suffer from the same defects of human nature as you and I and consequently can be expected to hang on to their cash cow with grim determination, even as they trip over the plain and obvious truth that it does not provide an adequate explanation for the initiation of the disease. Not to worry; the good news is that efforts are now under way to nail down a mitochondrial metabolic theory that *does* provide an adequate explanation for the initiation of cancer. Check.

## Obstacle #3: Flawed Research

The next big obstacle standing in the way of rooting out cancer relates to flawed research. In order to conduct research, you will need ready-made cancer cells. Currently, these are being marketed by Big Pharma. Referred to as "cell lines," the resurrected, reconstituted, neutered, stabilized, commercially homogenized cancer cells are packaged in Petri dishes and sold to research institutions at great profit.

The story of how one such cell line, dubbed "Hela cells," came to be commercially profitable is a tale that Big Pharma would rather sweep under a rug and not talk about. (Google *Hela cells*.) Initially, the cell line was said to have been named after a cancer patient called "Helen Lane" (a pejorative similar to "Jane Doe"). What came to light years later was that the cells were actually those of Henrietta Lacks, a thirty-one-year-old African American mother of five who died of cervical cancer at Johns Hopkins Hospital in Baltimore on October 4, 1951. Henrietta's name was not associated with the cell line until the news of it leaked in the 1970s. Apparently without Henrietta's knowledge, or her family's consent, her cancer cells have been a lucrative staple of the cancer industry for decades.

I see you shaking your head. I hear you say, "So what's wrong with that? If Henrietta's cells were perfectly suited for cancer research, preserving and marketing them to research institutions was the right thing to do, wasn't it?" Not quite. The problem with using cell lines in cancer research was explained in great detail by pathologist Dr. Gerald B. Dermer in his 1994 book, *The Immortal Cell.* It is the pathologist, not the researcher or the oncologist or even the surgeon, that determines if a tumor is malignant or benign. It is the pathologist who casts the final diagnostic decision, so you'd think that the opinion of one with a lifetime of experience looking at real cancer cells under a microscope would have carried a lot of weight back in 1994. Not so. Dermer's opinions, findings, and recommendations were dismissed, ignored, stonewalled, and at times, even scorned. Notwithstanding, he came very close to seeing the truth that the practitioners and purveyors of SMT have been tripping over ever since. He wrote the following thirty years ago:

> The one explanation that the experts will not consider, because it would invalidate a generation of research, is that the mutations are actually irrelevant to cancer initiation. The more mutations the experts discover, the more likely it becomes that all of them do not have the same importance. If any of the mutations are the *result* of cancer rather than its cause, the rest become suspect as well.[32]

The researcher is working with commercially homogenized cancer cells packed in Petri dishes (*in vitro*). The pathologist, on the other hand, is working with real cancer cells removed from a patient in a hospital (*in vivo*). Big difference, as Dermer points out:

> If we ever hope to win this war and make truly significant inroads against the modern scourge of cancer, the establishment must be willing to acknowledge its mistakes. Researchers must turn away from Petri dish "cancer" to the realities of human cancer. Four hundred years ago people were told that the sun moved around the earth. Today, the public understanding of cancer is just as inaccurate, for much the same reason: An incorrect

---

[32] Dr. Gerald B. Dermer, *The Immortal Cell* (New York, Avery Publishing Group, Inc., 1994), 75.

model of nature dominates the thought within an entire scientific field.[33]

You are shaking your head again. You are asking the same question: "What is so terribly wrong with using cancer cells conveniently packaged in Petri dishes to do research with?" Dermer answers your question:

> [O]n the bottom of a [Petri] dish, a lung tumor line looks like a breast tumor line, which looks like an ovarian tumor line, which looks like a prostate tumor line, etc., etc., ad infinitum. The differentiated features of the tumors are lost by the lines as they adapt to life under the artificial conditions of the culture environment. Cell lines show few of the signs of the differentiation that characterized their cellular ancestors because they have become undifferentiated (underdeveloped) in culture.[34]

Why do researchers continue to use *in vitro* cancer cells when they could be using *in vivo* cancer cells harvested from hospitals? Dermer answers this question as well:

> Malignant cells living in a tumor, just removed from a patient, are much more difficult to work with. Various types of normal cells are often present in a tumor, and the tumor itself remains alive for only a short period of time. It is difficult, if not impossible, to measure accurately the effects of experimental procedures on only the cancerous cells while they are alive. These difficulties slow the work and limit the kinds of experiments and analyses that can be performed. As a result, fewer papers are published by scientists who study [actual] tumors, than are published by [scientists who study] cell lines.[35]

---

[33] *ibid*, 10.

[34] *ibid*, 54

[35] *ibid*, 40

In research circles, there is an inside joke that goes something like this: "Papers are published to be counted, not to be read!" Face it; research grants are funded on the basis of the number of papers published. Imagine you are the CEO of one of the big pharmaceutical companies, and let me give you two choices: Do research using canned cancer cells, publish hundreds of papers, and receive billions in taxpayer funds; or do research using live cancer cells, publish just a few papers, and receive hardly anything by way of taxpayer funds. Which one would you choose? You see the problem. Every year, reams and reams of research papers get published. Every year, hundreds of thousands of Americans continue to die of cancer. All method and no content. All motion and no direction. All form and no substance.

Granted, you do run into difficulties when you try to conduct research using *in vivo* cancer cells harvested from hospitals. But those difficulties are no longer insurmountable. The difficulties that Dermer mentioned existed back in 1994 when he wrote *The Immortal Cell*. Biotechnology has come a long way since 1994. Given what biotech is capable of today, there is no reason why research should not be able to make the orderly transition from canned cancer cells to live cancer cells. *In vitro* canned cancer cells could still be used to train students in the procedures of research, but only to prepare them to graduate to the use of live cancer cells *in vivo*. Check.

## Obstacle #4: Vested Interests

i: Food and Beverage
ii: Pharmacological
iii: Chemical

The fourth obstacle standing in the way of rooting out cancer relates to the de-facto multibillion-dollar vested interests that various institutions have in the perpetuation of the disease. Be it from the foods involved; or the drugs involved; or the chemicals involved, wittingly or unwittingly, knowingly or unknowingly; they make money by contributing to the problem. Much like the relationship that exists between shark and remora, the relationship that exists between vested interests and the cancer industry can be summed up in the word *symbiosis*. Food-and-drug giants get rich making people sick, which makes the cancer industry get rich treating them after the fact. The two function like *symbionts* (creatures living together for mutual benefit).

Not to worry; this fourth obstacle can be removed using the "carrot and stick" approach. "Carrot and stick" refers to a combination of reward and punishment that can be used to encourage a stubborn beast of burden (or institution, or industry) to turn around and start moving in the right direction. People living in the underdeveloped areas of the world are familiar with the concept. They will tell you the quickest way to get that stubborn mule to move would be to dangle a carrot in front of his nose and whack him in the rear with a stick.

## How to Incentivize Food-and-Beverage Giants to Change Course

We have an aphorism of Hippocrates, the father of medicine, which is really a truism relating to health and disease:

"Let food be your medicine and medicine be your food."

Most of us don't have backyards to grow our own healthy foods in, much less acres of land to graze our own healthy livestock on. Not to worry; we can buy what we need from a supermarket. To their credit, food-and-beverage giants enable us to do that. Also to their credit, food-and-beverage giants provide gainful employment for millions. "Shutting them down," as some naïve young people suggest, would involve giving pink slips to millions in need of gainful employment. No need to shut down food-and-beverage giants. No need to throw the baby out with the bathwater. Just use the carrot and the stick to incentivize them to do the right thing instead.

In order to stay alive, people must eat food—meaning there will never be a shortage of demand for food. There will always be plenty of money to be made by providing people with healthy, nutritious, conveniently packaged, affordably priced foods. The demand will always be there, and, God permitting, the green earth will always provide the supply. Only the greed and depravity of man stands in the way of these two components coming together.

In order to remain viable in a universe such as this, people must eat food. But now, at long last, they are paying attention to *what* they eat. They are no longer going to feed their children foods that contain unhealthy ingredients. Consumers are waking up from the sleep of the dead! They are reading labels! The handwriting is on the wall! Institutions that insist on peddling unhealthy foods to humankind are about to be driven out of business by savvy consumers all over the world. The take-home message should be clear in all this: incentivize food-and-beverage giants to do the right thing! This way, they can stay in business, make lots of money—and continue to provide gainful employment for millions around the world. That's a win-win situation. Check.

## How to Incentivize Big Pharma to Change Course

The pharmaceutical corporations that manufacture cancer drugs are in business to make money. They, too, employ millions of people around the world—gifted, talented people who use their salaries to pay their mortgages, feed their children, cover expenses, and pay taxes. Clearly, it would not do to "shut down" Big Pharma, as some unthinking young people seem to want to do. Shutting down Big Pharma would involve giving pink slips to millions of gainfully employed people.

Yes, Big Pharma has made lots of mistakes, but mistakes are often preludes to progress. Winston Churchill once said, "All men make mistakes, but only wise men learn from their mistakes." Think of how many lessons had to be learned (and how many mistakes had to be made) before the drug penicillin came online. Think of how many lives have been saved by the use of penicillin. Did pharmaceutical companies make money from penicillin? Yes, and rightfully so.

Big Pharma has made lots of mistakes—and learned lots of valuable lessons. Big Pharma is now in possession of vast databases relating to the effectiveness of thousands of drugs with different applications—some preventative, some palliative, some curative, some therapeutic, some analgesic. Any way you look at it, this is a wealth of information, a priceless resource for millennials to build on. The current problem with Big Pharma is that it is always looking for the holy grail of chemotherapy—the alchemist's gold; the elusive brew; the miracle blend; the magic bullet; the all-powerful, all-inclusive, universal, "wide spectrum" poison that will kill cancer overnight and make billions for its manufacturer. This is a pipe dream. It is the delusion that has sidetracked researchers into chasing their own tails for decades.

Up to now, the cancer drugs Big Pharma has been marketing have been geared to the somatic mutation theory of cancer (SMT), a theory with more holes in it than Swiss cheese. Replacing SMT with a mitochondrial metabolic theory (MMT) will create the need for a whole new range of pharmacological solutions. The paradigm shift from SMT to MMT will create the need for a broad range of new drugs that could be used, for example, to target the glucose and glutamine fuels that cancer needs to survive, grow, and metastasize (see Chapter 18 of Seyfried's magnum opus *Cancer as a Metabolic Disease* for more on this).

So then, here also, the take-home message should be clear. No need to shut down Big Pharma. No need to throw the baby out with the bathwater. Just incentivize Big Pharma to change course instead. In this way, pharma can do the right thing, continue to make lots of money—and employ tens of thousands of gifted scientists, researchers, physicists, chemists, and lab assistants around the world, working together to rid the world of the plague of the twentieth century. Check.

## How to Incentivize Chemical Giants to Change Course

Recently, a jury in Oakland, California, ordered chemical giant Monsanto to pay $2 billion in damages to a couple whose cancer was linked to the pesticide Roundup. Numerous other Roundup lawsuits are now in the works. Has Monsanto learned any lessons from its alleged mistakes? Is it going to see the light and change its ways? Or is it going to legally-pigally continue with business as usual?

Here also, the take-home message should be clear. No need to shut down Monsanto. No need to throw the baby out with the bathwater. Just use the carrot and the stick to incentivize the chemical giant to do the right thing instead. This way it, too, can stay in business, make lots of money, help the farmers of the world feed all the families of the earth—and continue to provide gainful employment for millions. Check.

## Carrot and Stick

Removing the obstacles listed above can be done using the "carrot and stick" stratagem. Carrot, stick, and wise legislation can require the orderly, gradual phasing out of unhealthy foods, harmful drugs, and toxic chemicals. The carrot would relate to the rewards of an ample subsistence earned in a free market. The stick would relate to transparency, public accountability, and rules with severe consequences. No more legally-pigally. No more hiding behind an army of fancy-shmancy lawyers clad in Armani suits and smelling of French cologne. No more turning a blind eye to the fly in the ointment of American democracy. Institutions that persist in making money by wrecking the health of humankind will face consequences they will no longer be able to plan for, avoid, avert, afford, or work around, slush fund or no slush fund. Check.

## The Fly in the Ointment of Democracy

In a democracy such as ours, reform begins with public accountability. We need only to glance at our own history to see that this is so. More than one hundred United States Congresses have investigated and exposed every form of impropriety, malfeasance, iniquity, and injustice to the light of public accountability. There have been election scandals and investigations of questionable practices of railroads, oil, transportation, agriculture, food-and-drug, insurance, shipping, steel, coal, housing, communications, and utilities companies. From Teapot Dome to Watergate to Fast and Furious, almost everything that affects the health, well-being, and pocketbook of the American family has at various times been opened up to the light of public scrutiny. Through it all, however, a handful of institutions have managed to evade public accountability. How does this happen in a "democracy" such as ours?

It happens because lobbyists are allowed to roam the corridors of Capitol Hill. Who are these influence peddlers? What are they up to? What do they want? To find out, just follow the money trail. Follow the bread crumbs all the way from the boardrooms of vested interests to K-Street in Washington, DC, and from there, to the hallowed halls of the United States Congress right next door. How much money are these lobbyists being paid to invade the inner sanctum of our government and browbeat our elected officials into supporting the interests of their big bosses? Does anyone in Congress know? Does anyone in Congress care? To give just one example, fifty years ago, the sugar lobby paid pseudo-scientists money to come up with phony data downplaying the effects of refined white sugar on human health. (Google "The sugar lobby paid scientists … ") This sort of rotten business is just the tip of the iceberg, and it has to stop. The incestuous marriage between K-Street and the United States Congress must be annulled in due process of law. K-Street's access to the processes of government must be limited in scope and dimension to what Congress deems "appropriate." Check.

## Obstacle #5: Uninformed Public

Reflecting on the words of Hippocrates, "Let food be your medicine and medicine be your food," the other great obstacle that stands in the way of rooting out cancer relates to a planetwide dearth of information about the causes of health and disease. Of the billions of educated people on earth, how many do you think have as much as heard of "mitochondria"? How many do you think have heard of "**ATP**"? How many do you think can connect the dots between free energy and health? How many do you think can connect the dots between impaired **ATP** production and disease? How many? A handful? Let us agree that this is a big part of the problem. Ignorance is not bliss. Ignorance is pathological, literally carcinogenic in this case.

## How to Educate Consumers about Health and Nutrition

The millennial mandate of rooting out cancer within twenty-five years will require educating all the families of the earth about (A) the body's specific energy needs and (B) the *quality* and *quantity* of foods needed to meet those requirements (emphasis on *quality and quantity*). A planetwide education such as this will no doubt have the added effect of killing two birds with one stone. It goes without saying that the quickest way to stop food-and-beverage giants from infusing the meat of humankind with harmful steroids or adulterating the drink of humankind with "high-fructose" abominations would be to educate consumers about the long-term effects of such compounds.

If we are *serious* about making the world a cancer-free place to live and prosper in, we must encourage all the families of the earth to *stop* patronizing the purveyors of the disease. We must encourage all the families of the earth to *stop* buying the colorfully packaged, cleverly advertised, overprocessed, overemulsified, sugar-coated, artificially sweetened, additive-loaded, chemically hydrogenated, genetically altered, nutritionally mutilated, "crispy, chewy, gooey, crunchy, tasty" junk foods that impair mitochondrial function. *Stop already!* Read the label, for God's sake! Read it with a magnifying glass if you have to! Stop patronizing the producers of unhealthy foods, and they will stop producing them. Check.

## Obstacle #6: Money, Finances, and Revenue

It's going to take a lot of money to root out cancer within twenty-five years. For starters, it will be up to you millennials to persuade the United States Congress to *stop* wasting billions of taxpayer dollars on flawed science and ineffective research. Don't be shy about how you go about doing this. Your right "to petition the Government for a redress of grievance" is guaranteed by the First Amendment of the United States Constitution. Don't hesitate to exercise that right. Flood the offices of Congressional Budget Offices with your petitions day and night. Keep flooding them until results are forthcoming.

Everyone on earth is ready to support you! Everyone on earth is anxious to root out cancer. Everyone on earth is happy to part with money to that end. Unfortunately, most of the money that people so cheerfully part with ends up in the coffers of flawed science and ineffective research. You can't root out cancer that way. You will bounce off the same walls and end up right back where you started. The flawed science that is perpetuating cancer has to be replaced with real science; otherwise, we might as well admit defeat, throw in the towel, and learn to live with the insidious disease.

## How to Make Acquisition of Funds

I see you shaking your head again. You are saying, "Taxpayers are already buried up to their eyebrows in private and public debt, so where is all that money going to come from?" Not to worry; with the creation of a global GoFundMe account and a little help from the rich and famous, removing the sixth obstacle should not be too difficult. Illustrious billionaires such as Elon Musk, founder of Tesla and SpaceX, must be doggedly pestered to the point of releasing the needed funds. Many of these illustrious billionaires are already involved in praiseworthy causes of their own, and it will be to their credit to go down in history as the ones that helped finance mankind's epic battle against cancer. Check.

## Revenue

Don't worry about the money; it will show up in due course. The thing to worry about is *revenue.* Question: Why does the cancer establishment continue to do the same thing and expect a different result? Answer: Because of the *revenue* it brings in! Billions of dollars in *revenue!* To date, the business models that bring in all that *revenue* are built around the somatic mutation theory of cancer (SMT), a theory with more holes in it than Swiss cheese. The replacement of SMT with a mitochondrial metabolic theory (MMT) will require a new business model that can provide adequate levels of *revenue* for hospitals, physicians, clinics, and health-care workers; otherwise, the transition from SMT to MMT will remain a pipe dream.

## How to Create a New Business Model

Creating the new business model will require the talents of visionaries like Dr. Martin Makary, for example. A surgeon with professorship at Johns Hopkins Medical Center, Marty Makary has a long history of doing hand-to-hand combat with cancer. His recent *New York Times* bestselling business book of the year, *The Price We Pay—What Broke American Health Care and How to Fix It*, is nothing short of an indictment of our health-care system. The contents of this book will shock you to the core of your being. Wanton waste of public monies; unconscionable overcharging of procedures; a veritable orgy of price gauging; incestuous relationships between "pharmacy benefit managers" (PBMs), insurance companies, hospitals, and physicians ... the list goes on an on. To say that our health-care system is broken would be the understatement of the century! In reading Marty's book, your author reached the point where he had to put it down and go for a walk, literally feeling nauseous. Makary and his team of researchers deserve a Nobel Prize for ferreting out the truth and raking in the muck. Read the book for yourself and see if it doesn't make you want to utter a scream of profound agony.

The gloom and doom notwithstanding, Dr. Makary closes on a positive note that resonates with the audience of this publication—millennials and younger generation:

> Most meaningful has been the greatest gift a university professor could ever receive—being inspired by the many young people who have told me they are committed to working on these issues at their hospital, university, or business. If you know the millennial mindset, you know that these young people want to be a part of something larger than themselves ... They want to change the world.[36]

## Obstacle #7: Loss of Momentum

The critical path to rooting out cancer within twenty-five years will require *sustained* effort throughout the length and breadth of a quarter of a century. Naturally, the baton will have to be passed along in due time, from Generation Y (millennials) to Generations Z and possibly Alpha. Meaning now and then, there may be a discontinuity in the critical path, a tendency to slack off, take things for granted and lose momentum. To avoid the existential pitfall, the incumbent generation (millennials) must create a *matrix* and a *metric* that will (A) ensure sustained momentum throughout the twenty-five-year period and (B) gauge success or failure at each step of the way. By *matrix*, we mean an organizational structure designed to

---

[36] Marty Makary, MD, *The Price We Pay* (New York, NY, Bloomsbury Publishing, 2019), 254-55.

keep the critical path *moving* in the right direction. By *metric*, we mean an analytical tool, a key performance indicator (KPI) that will look at the whole landscape of the critical path and provide accurate assessments of performance or nonperformance at any point in time. Check.

# Chapter 17

# Critical Path Benchmarks

A journey of a thousand miles begins with a single step.
—Chinese proverb

Free energy is what the cells of our bodies need to perform the *work* of keeping us alive and healthy in a universe such as this. Free energy in the form of **ATP** is synthesized by mitochondria swimming around in the cytoplasm of our cells. If we are serious about making the world a cancer-free place for all the families of the earth to live and prosper in, it only remains for us to ensure mitochondrial vitality, potency, and functionality. This can be done via two steps:

> **Step 1:** All foods, additives, drugs, medications, hygiene products, toiletries, cosmetics, chemicals, pesticides, and compounds that enter the human body must be assessed for their effects on mitochondrial function.

> **Step 2:** All foods, additives, drugs, medications, hygiene products, toiletries, cosmetics, chemicals, pesticides, and compounds shown to impair mitochondrial function *to the extent of the impairment* must be phased out in an orderly manner and replaced with substitutes that do not impair mitochondrial function.

This doesn't have to be done overnight; neither does it have to be done in a manner that places undue burdens on human economies. It has to be done nevertheless, if we are *serious* about rooting out cancer and not just talking about it—"yada, yada, blah, blah, blah!" Question: Are we *serious* about rooting out cancer? Yes or no? If the answer is yes, then let's get off the fence, roll up our sleeves, put our shoulders to the wheel, and just do it. If the answer is no, presumably because we don't want to upset the apple cart of the *revenue* that cancer brings in, then let's get off the fence, admit defeat, throw in the towel and just learn to live with the insidious disease. Either way, let's get off the fence, make up our minds, and go with the decision.

Rooting out cancer within twenty-five years won't be easy, but nothing worthwhile is. Yes, there will be pushback from vested interests. Yes, there will legally-pigally, finger pointing, name calling, *ad hominem*, mudslinging, sloganeering, cant, propaganda, invectives—"Health Gestapo! Health Gestapo! Food police! Food police!" Not to worry; unless given over to reprobate minds, the CEOs, directors, and stockholders of the cancer industry would want their children and grandchildren to live in a cancer-free world as well, so take their Chicken Little "the sky is falling" remonstrations with a grain of salt and keep plugging away, one step at a time, steady as she goes, "with malice toward none and good will toward all."

Without presuming to dictate the specifics of the critical path, the following may be used as a skeletal framework that can be perfected along the way.

## First Benchmark (Years 1–5)

### Millennial Council

A council of sorts will be needed to oversee the entire landscape of the critical path. Borrowing something from George Lucas's *Star Wars,* major decisions could be made by a higher-level "Jedi Council" and carried out by lower-level "Padawans" (interns). This higher-level council would have to be composed of uniquely qualified individuals hailing from related fields of science, medicine, academia, technology, nutrition, geopolitics, economy, and finance. To qualify to sit on the Millennial Council, these "Master Jedi" would have to demonstrate that they have *no* vested interests in disease in general, cancer in particular. Check.

## Cancer Clock

A "Cancer Clock" will have to be created to count down the twenty-five years (216,000 days) backwards, providing all the families of the earth with a constant reminder of what's at stake, how much has been accomplished, and how much remains to be done before time runs out. The ticking of the Cancer Clock will also encourage you millennials to take nothing for granted; stay on course; maintain momentum; daily prioritize to-do lists; undertake day-end reviews of "done," "carry forward," etc.; building confidence as you stay on course and forge ahead, come what may.

The creation of the Cancer Clock would call for a globally televised/streamed ceremony in which a noteworthy person of your choice would press a big, red button and start it ticking. Suggestion: in honor of beloved Steve Jobs, who died of cancer on October 5, 2011, Tim Cook, current CEO of Apple, would be a good candidate. Check.

## Tempus Fugit

No time to waste. Assume that the clock is already ticking, and get to work. ASAP, bring together talent from all over the world to start assessing the effects of all foods, additives, drugs, medications, hygiene products, toiletries, cosmetics, chemicals, pesticides, and compounds on mitochondrial function. Bring together scientific talent relating to bioenergetics of the human body; academic talent relating to experimental procedures; chemical talent relating to pharmacology; nutritional talent relating healthy foods; biotech talent relating to cell biology; technological talent relating to cutting-edge diagnostic tools; and economic talent relating to the implementation of the MMT business model.

## Guiding Principle

No need to complicate things. No need to go overboard. No need to go to extremes. No need to engage in diatribes and *ad hominem*. No need to get personal about anything. No need to point Manichaean fingers at people. Keep it simple, stick to the issues, and keep plugging away, one step at a time, steady as she goes, "with malice towards none, and good will towards all." Always remember: "Principles, not people; the sin, not the sinner."

## General Plan

Avoiding specific brand names, all compounds that enter the human body can be broken down into groupings and their effects on mitochondrial function investigated experimentally. Examples of groupings follow. These can be changed, modified, added to, corrected, and updated as necessary. (I may have misplaced some categories, and others could easily overlap.)

## Foods

- Whole foods (no ingredients)
- Processed foods (additives and ingredients)
- Meats
- Lipids
- Dairy
- Carbohydrates
- Grains
- Glutens
- Cereals
- Salt
- Sugar
- Flour
- Supplements
- Treats
- Snacks
- Caffeine
- Other categories?

## Food Additives

- Nutritional
- Bulk enhancement
- Processing

➤ Preservatives
➤ Hormonal (livestock, poultry)
➤ Sensory agents
➤ Other categories?

## Drugs and Medications

➤ Preventative
➤ Palliative
➤ Curative
➤ Therapeutic
➤ Analgesic
➤ Antibiotic
➤ Stimulants
➤ Anti-Depressants
➤ Statins
➤ Beta blockers
➤ Calcium blockers
➤ Blood thinners
➤ Hallucinogens
➤ Dissociatives
➤ Opioids
➤ Inhalants
➤ Other categories?

## Hygiene Products, Toiletries, Cosmetics

➤ Used to wash the body
➤ Used to wash hair
➤ Used to clean teeth
➤ Used for shaving
➤ Used for odor suppression
➤ Used for hygiene
➤ Used for cosmetics
➤ Other categories?

## Chemicals

- PFAS (e.g., nonstick coatings)
- Detergents
- Antimicrobials
- Disinfectants
- Flame retardants
- BPA (bisphenols)
- Phthalates (plastics)
- Alcohol
- Nicotine
- Tobacco products
- Solvents
- Lubricants
- Oils
- Metals
- Other categories?

## Pesticides

- Insecticides
- Herbicides
- Rodenticides
- Bactericides
- Fungicides
- Larvicides
- Other categories?

Mitochondria can be grown in cell culture, and the short-term, accumulative, and long-term effects of compounds on their function can be observed under TEMs (transmitting electron microscopes that reveal changes in *internal structures*) and SEMs (scanning electron microscopes that reveal changes in *surface structures*). Other than the availability of TEMs and SEMs, this should pose no problem, as most major universities have their own, and those that don't can be equipped as such (at a cost of about $60,000 a piece); or they can participate via the worldwide Shared Instrumentation Network.

## Baseline Acquisition

In Chapter 5, we discussed the relationship between free energy and structure and surmised the two to be somewhat fungible—that is, of such constitution that a part or quantity of one could be replaced by a part or quantity of the other. If this is true, then you would expect to find equivalence between mitochondrial *structure* and mitochondrial *function*. The element of fungibility would look something like this:

$$\text{Structure} \leftrightarrow \text{Function} \leftrightarrow \text{Structure}$$

Great architects have always differed on the question about form and function, some arguing, "form follows function," and others insisting, "function follows form." Famous architect Frank Lloyd Wright is thought to have put the controversy to rest by saying this: "Form and function should be one, joined in a spiritual union" (1908, unverified). We may be dealing with a similar dichotomy here. Does mitochondrial form follow mitochondrial function, or does mitochondrial function follow mitochondrial form? Or are the two "as one, joined in a spiritual union"? What do you think?

Either way, given the element of fungibility, one would expect impaired mitochondrial function to correspond with impaired mitochondrial structure, and vice versa. In other words, we would expect normal mitochondria to exhibit normal structures and abnormal mitochondria to exhibit abnormal structures. But how would we know the difference between the two? I mean, what are normal mitochondrial organelles supposed to look like, anyway? If we don't know what normal mitochondria are supposed to look like, how are we going to tell the difference between normal and abnormal, given that mitochondria come in many different sizes and shapes? (Google "mitochondrial images.")

We can reasonably assume, for example, that environmental toxins can impair mitochondrial structures. But what would the impaired structures look like? Would their basic shapes differ from those of normal mitochondria? If so, in what way, and to what extent? Would their surface structures appear distorted? Would their internal structures appear distorted? Would they be missing something by way of *cristae* (folds in their inner membranes that increase surface area), mtDNA, or ribosomes? Unless we have an extensive database relating to what normal mitochondria are supposed to look like, we will have no basis for analyzing the effects of toxic chemicals on their structure/function. What we need is a "plumb line" that will enable us to distinguish between straight and crooked, so to speak, a baseline database (perhaps consisting of computer-enhanced electron micrographs) that will enable us to distinguish between normal and damaged mitochondrial organelles. With the acquisition of such a database, we will then be in a position to investigate the effects of compounds on mitochondrial structure and function. Check.

## Worldwide Collaboration

The preliminaries notwithstanding, the plan of action would not be complicated at all. The task of assessing the effects of compounds on mitochondrial function could be divided up between the 20,000+ universities around the world. These would be called upon to undertake the same experiments using the same samples, their findings shared among all. Findings could be published along following lines (these are grossly oversimplified):

- **Category Name** (e.g., Phthalates)
- **Short-term effects on mitochondria:**
  - Negligible ☐
  - Mild ☐
  - Moderate ☐
  - Significant ☐
  - Severe ☐

- **Accumulative effects on mitochondria:**
  - Negligible ☐
  - Mild ☐

> o   Moderate ☐
> o   Significant ☐
> o   Severe ☐

> ➤ **Long terms effects on mitochondria:**
> o   Negligible ☐
> o   Mild ☐
> o   Moderate ☐
> o   Significant ☐
> o   Severe ☐

> ➤ **Recommendation(s)** ______________

Dividing the task between 20,000+ universities would not only speed up the process, but would also stand a good chance of weeding out false readings. Say, if a certain university in one part of the world were to assess the effects of endocrine disruptors on mitochondria to be mild but a multitude of universities elsewhere were to assess it to be severe, the former would be called upon to go over its finding and/or repeat the experiment with a view toward investigating the source of the discrepancy. (The stuff of the scientific discipline, if you catch my drift.) Check.

## Second Benchmark (Years 5–10)

### Implementation of the Findings of the First Benchmark

All chemicals shown to impair mitochondrial function, *to the extent of the impairment,* will have to be phased out in a gradual fashion, or replaced with substitutes that do not impair mitochondrial function. Naturally, those classified as severe would have to be phased out sooner than those classified as mild. Some would not have to be phased out at all. Here is a rudimentary example: a certain chemical in a household compound of chemicals, say a shampoo, has been found to impair mitochondrial function. Do we need phase out all shampoos? No, we just need to replace the suspect chemical with one that does not impair mitochondrial function, and ladies could continue to shampoo their beautiful hair. I'm oversimplifying, but you catch my drift.

The twenty-five-year critical path to rooting out cancer will concomitantly require the bringing together of qualified people from all over the world, including religious leaders respecting the God-given rights of man; ethical leaders respecting the value of a single human life; legal experts respecting international law; geopolitical experts respecting the rights of sovereign nations; mediators respecting coordination between governmental health authorities; and economic experts respecting the effects of phase-outs on human economies, employment, and inflation. The effects of phase-outs on human economies, employment, and inflation could in turn be mitigated by financial assistance from the International Monetary Fund, debt relief from the World Bank, allowances from the World Trade Organization, grants, tax write-offs, subsidies, and government incentives similar to those afforded by the Covid-19 response and recovery conventions of 2020. Check.

## Third Benchmark (Years 10–15)

There are to be determined, pursuant to accomplishments of the first and second benchmarks. This will become evident as you stay on course and "peel away the layers of the onion." Always remember: "if it can't be measured, it's not progress."

## Fourth Benchmark (Years 15–20)

There are to be determined, pursuant to accomplishments of the first, second, and third benchmarks. This, too, will become evident as you stay on course and continue to "peel away the layers of the onion." Always remember: "if it can't be measured, it's not progress."

## Fifth Benchmark (Years 20–25)

The completion of the fifth and final benchmark will mark the calendar of the world with the auspicious year in which the sons of Adam and daughters of Eve succeeded in evicting the devil of cancer from the premises of the planet. The author is fully persuaded that the goal *will* be accomplished, and the date will be commemorated by generations for years to come. It will be celebrated by festivities including solemn acts of thanksgiving to God; ringing of church bells; blowing of shofars; drum rolls; pomp and circumstance; victory parades; fanfare; lights; fireworks; singing and dancing in the streets—spontaneous outbreaks of joy and gladness from one end of the earth to the other.

# Afterword
## Of Interest to Ecclesiastic and Rabbinic Scholars

The Bible was written in pre-scientific ages in which our Heavenly Father had to use the language of accommodation to convey great truths to us; among them:

- The ontology of the cosmos (Genesis 1:1)
- The anthropology of man (Genesis 2:7)
- The relationship between the ontology of the cosmos and the anthropology of man (1 John 2:16)
- The tendency of the anthropology of man to come into alignment with the ontology of the cosmos (Romans 12:2)
- The tendency of humankind to want to go with the universal flow toward more and more probable states (Proverbs 14:12)
- The love of God manifesting in His prohibitions against going with the universal flow towards more and more probable states (Exodus 20:2–17)
- The love of God manifesting in the gift of salvation offered to all who have gone with the universal flow, are willing to confess to having does so, and are prepared change course (John 3:16)

In pre-scientific ages, the Bible had to use imagery, anthropomorphisms, allegories, similes, metaphors, illustrations, analogies, and parables to convey these great truths to us. In lieu of the universal principle that discriminates against the unstable complexity of life (aka increasing entropy), we find the Bible positing a corresponding principality (principle enforcer) and calling it "the adversary" (in Hebrew, *ha satan*). By positing the principality in lieu of the principle, our Heavenly Father was able efficiently to caution all the families of the earth about the spiritual and moral pitfalls thereof (Galatians 6:8). Humankind, created in the image of God (Genesis 1:27), yet formed from the physics of the universe (Genesis 2:7), may still be unaware of the spiritual pitfalls associated with the universal principle of increasing entropy, but by now, all the inhabitants of the earth have heard of something called "devil."

## "Satan"

If we believe the Bible to be the inspired Word of God, we may be sure that its Divine Author has been careful about the use of words, clearly dividing between common and proper nouns. Examples of common nouns would be: *the* butcher, *the* baker, *the* candle maker, *the* doctor, *the* lawyer, *the* thief, *the* enemy, *the* adversary. Examples of proper nouns would be names such as Tom, Dick, Harry, Tina, Deborah, and Sarah. The Hebrew expression *ha satan* ("*the* adversary") was initially preceded by the definite article *ha* ("*the*"), rendering it into a common noun. Somewhere along the line, however, *ha satan* (common noun) metamorphosed into the "Satan" (name) that most Christians believe in today. How did that happen?

## Dualism

Belief in dualism, it seems, has been a fixture of history since time immemorial. Two opposing deities. Two contrary and coeternal principles. Two antipodes of light and darkness. Good God versus bad God. Good guys versus bad guys. The dark side of the force versus the light side. In ancient Egypt, it was used to denounce enemies as "children of darkness." In ancient Persia, it took on cosmic proportions to invade diverse religions and cultures. By the time of Christ, it had assumed apocalyptic dimensions in the ranks of the Qumran Sect. Later on in the Christian era, it assumed Gnostic, Manichaean, Bogomilian, and Cathar forms. In the mercifully brief period preceding the Second World War, it reared up its ugly head in terms of national socialism ("Our race *uber alles!*"). Belief in dualism is still with us today, most notably in some regions of the Middle East, and, most regrettably, in many Christian churches. How did that happen? How could so many of our churches have allowed themselves to become mired in a pagan doctrine that dates back to dualism of Zoroaster?

## Zoroaster's Dualism

The prophet Zoroaster, thought to have come on the Persian scene around 660 BC, was among the first to model the universe after a Manichaean struggle between good and evil, that is, between the adherents of the good god "Ahura Mazda" and the minions of the evil god "Ahriman." With the expansion of the Persian Empire circa 500 BC, Zoroaster's dualism invaded the core and substance of diverse cultures as far as the Danube on the west and the Indus River on the east, the Sudan on the south and the Caucasus on the north.

Regardless of what Zoroaster had in mind when he modeled the universe after a proto-Manichaean struggle between two coequal "primal spirits" (Zoroaster's religious opus, *Avesta*, yasna 30.1–6, 8–9), in the centuries that followed, his dualism grew into a bogeyman of worldwide proportions. Human nature, looking for an excuse to demonize "others" competing for the same resources, found what it was looking for in religious, racial and cultural animus.

It is said that Zoroaster's dualism has exerted more influence in history than many other religions combined. Circa 510 B.C. the Jews of the southern kingdom of Judah were taken captive into Babylon/Persia, where some of them assimilated the dualism and later brought it back with them to Jerusalem under Ezra and Nehemiah. Cyrus the Great's edict, recorded in Ezra 1:1–4, allowed returning Jews to rebuild the temple and restore their biblical traditions. Howbeit their seventy-year sojourn in Babylon/Persia had cost them something in terms of *syncretism* (cross-pollination of cultures, blending of traditions, watering down of doctrines). In his opus titled *The Other God,* Yuri Stoyanov comments on one aspect of that syncretism:

> While, however, the Iranian influences in the New Testament are still keenly debated, it is beyond doubt that the Christian concept of the devil as the head of the realm of evil and originator of sin and death was

determined by the radical transformations in Jewish notions of evil and Satan in the centuries that followed the dramatic vicissitudes that transformed and left their lasting imprint on the Jewish world in the sixth century BC—the Babylonian Captivity and return to Zion.[37]

The Jews that went into Babylonian captivity took with them the Biblical concept of *ha satan*. The Jews that returned from Babylonian captivity brought with them the Persianized, personal "Satan" that most Christians believe in today. The doctrinal alteration is born out by two different accounts of the taking of the census of Israel by David:

> **2 Samuel 24:1:** And again the anger of the Lord was kindled against Israel, and He incited David against them to say, "Go, number Israel and Judah."

> **1 Chronicles 21:1:** And Satan stood up against Israel, and enticed David to take a census of the people of Israel.

Is the Bible contradicting itself? How come in Second Samuel, it is God who is telling David to take a census of the people of Israel, but in First Chronicles, it is "Satan" who is telling him to do that? The explanation of course is that Second Samuel was written before the Babylonian/Persian captivity, whereas First Chronicles was written during or after. Obviously, some Jewish ideas about the devil had gotten mixed up with the Persian one, prompting the Divine Author of the Bible to place, as it were, a flashing red light in First Chronicles 21:1, as though to say "Caution! Caution!"

## Manichaean vs Augustinian Devil

Humankind may still be in the dark about the way in which the ontology of the universe orients the anthropology of man towards spiritually destructive ends, but by now, all the families of the earth have an

---

[37] Yuri Stoyanov, *The Other God* (London: Yale Nota Bene, Yale University Press, 2000), 2.

intuitive apprehension regarding some "devil" behind the scenes, so to speak. Question: Would such a "devil" be Manichaean or Augustinian? Mathematician and philosopher Norbert Weiner (1894-1964) tackled the question decades ago:

> The scientist is always working to discover the order and organization of the universe, and is thus playing a game against the arch enemy, disorganization. Is this devil Manichaean or Augustinian? Is it a contrary force opposed to order or is it the very absence of order itself? … The Manichaean devil is an opponent, like any other opponent, who is determined on victory and will use any trick of craftiness or dissimulation to obtain victory … On the other hand, the Augustinian devil, which is not a power in itself, but the measure of our own weakness, may require our full resources to uncover, but when we have uncovered it, we have in a certain sense exorcised it. …[38]

The Manichaean devil that most Christians believe in is a *person*. The Augustinian devil, on the other hand, is not a person at all. I see you shaking your head. I hear you say, "What does Augustine have to do with any of this?" Well, as it turns out, Augustine has a great deal to do with what we are talking about here. By defining evil as *privatio boni* ("privation of good"), Augustine rendered evil into something insubstantial and the author thereof into something impersonal.

An illustration might be sought to clear up any confusion that may exist regarding Augustine's definition of evil as *privatio boni*. Let us imagine that we are somewhere in the darkness of deep space, far from sources of light. Stated figuratively, unless someone comes along and turns on a light, darkness will be selected automatically. Why? Because darkness is the natural norm, apart from which there is nothing else to select. Out there, darkness would be the *default* state, and light would be the exception to the rule. Does this mean that darkness is a thing? No, darkness is not a thing. Darkness is merely "the absence of light" (*privatio lux*), just as evil

---

[38] Norbert Wiener, *The Human Use of Human Beings* (New York, Da Capo Press, Inc. 1954), 34–36.

is "the absence of good" (*privatio boni*). Let's take a look at the opening passages of God's Book:

> In the beginning God created the heavens and the earth. The earth was without form, and void; and darkness was on the face of the deep. ... (Genesis 1:1–2)

Is the Bible telling us that void and darkness are "things"? Of course not. Void and darkness represent the *absence* of things about to be created:

> And God said, Let there be light: and there was light. (Genesis 1:2–3)

Light can be said to be a "thing." Darkness cannot. Light "is" (has a property). Darkness "is not" (has no property). So then, to arrive at an understanding of Augustine's definition of evil as *privatio boni*, all we have to do is extrapolate the relationship between light and darkness to the relationship between good and evil. Remove the light, and darkness will be selected by default. Remove the good, and evil will be selected by default. This, in principle, is what the Bible has been warning about all along. This, in effect, is what the Irish Statesman Edmund Burke had in mind when he made that famous statement of his, "The only thing necessary for the triumph of evil is for good men to do nothing."

## Manichaean Devil

As to who or what this personal, Manichaean devil is supposed to be, your author can find no better description than the one that he ran into in the doctrinal statement of faith he was asked to sign prior to taking a course in hermeneutics at a local church. The statement reads as follows:

> **Paragraph XI. Satan**
> We believe there is a real personal devil of great malevolence, cunning, and power, who seeks to deceive, tempt, kill, steal and destroy, yet his power is limited by God to only what God permits him to do ...

These words describe one of the core beliefs of churchgoers today. "Satan," the antipode of God, is a cunning and powerful *person* who is able freely to run around the world, deceiving, tempting, killing, stealing, and destroying at will—with God's permission. I dare say, you will not find a single orthodox rabbi on earth who would agree with a Manichaean construct such as this. Yet, many rabbis would, perhaps, agree with an Augustinian construct whereby God would grant unrepentant sinners their wish by allowing them to follow the natural impulse (Hebrew, *yetzer ha ra*) to go with the universal flow toward more and more probable states, culminating in sin and death (Proverbs 14:12, Romans 1:28).

## "Fallen Angel"

Ask a hundred Christians what this personal, Manichaean devil is supposed to be, and ninety-nine of them will say, "He is a fallen angel!" The belief that the devil is a fallen angel is not supported by the testimony of the Bible itself:

> [I]f God spared not the angels that sinned, but cast them down to hell, and delivered them into chains of darkness, to be reserved unto judgment ... (2 Peter 2:4)

> And the angels who did not keep their proper domain, but left their own abode, He [God] has reserved in everlasting chains under darkness for the judgment of the great day. (Jude 1:6)

If God has reserved the fallen angels in "everlasting chains" waiting for "judgment of the great day," then who or what is this Manichaean devil that is running around the world "deceiving, tempting, killing, stealing, and destroying?"

## "Lucifer"

The Hebrew appellation *heylel* (Strong's Hebrew 1966, "shining one"), rendered "Lucifer" in English Bibles, is assumed by most Christians to refer to the personal devil that they were brought up to believe in. Concerning the grave error on which the assumption stands, let me only say this: if you, dear reader, were brought up to believe that the passages in Isaiah 14:12 and Ezekiel 28:11–19 confirm your belief in a personal devil called "Lucifer," I strongly encourage you to read the careful analysis of both passages by Dr. Craig Keener, professor of biblical studies at Asbury Seminary in Kentucky. They can found at these websites: https://craigkeener.com/does-isaiah-1412-14-refer-to-lucifers-fall-from-heaven/ and https://craigkeener.com/does-ezekiel-2812-14-refer-to-the-devil/

## The Book of Job

The oldest book in the Bible, Job is a rich repository of all the biblical genres we study when we take a course in hermeneutics. Superb narrative, cosmic imagery, divine law, lofty wisdom, piercing dialogue, exquisite poetry, implied prophecy, it is all in all a superlative exposition of the purpose of God in (A) creating a universe in which we will all face challenges and (B) how to partner with our Heavenly Father to overcome those challenges. It is in this enlarged context that we run into a civil discourse between God and *ha satan* (Job 1:6–12).

As the narrative goes, on a day when "the sons of God" (mistranslated "angels" is some Bibles) come to give accounts of themselves, the principality *ha satan* also shows up to give an account of himself. God asks him where he's coming from, and *ha satan* responds, "From going to and fro on the earth, and from walking back and forth on it" (Job 1:7).

> Then the Lord said to Satan, "Have you considered My servant Job, that there is none like him on the earth, a blameless and upright man, one who fears God and shuns evil?" (Job 1:8)

The devil finds fault with proposition:

> So Satan answered the Lord and said, "Does Job fear God for nothing? Have You not made a hedge around him, around his household, and around all that he has on

every side? You have blessed the work of his hands, and his possessions have increased in the land. But now, stretch out Your hand and touch all that he has, and he will surely curse You to Your face!" (Job 1:10)

In trying to understand the narrative, we must lay aside the traditions of men and go back to the fundamentals of the Word of God:

And the Lord God formed man of the dust of the ground, and breathed into his nostrils the breath of life; and man became a living being. (Genesis 2:7)

God formed man from the dust of the ground (the physics of the universe). When the "serpent" persuaded Adam and Eve to give the primacy to the dust of their constitution, instead of God, God relegated the dominion of the serpent to that of dust:

[U]pon thy belly shalt thou go, and dust shalt thou eat all the days of thy life. (Genesis 3:14, KJV)

Given the imagery, the devil's complaint might go something like this:

➤ You, God, formed Job from the dust of the ground.
➤ You, God, decreed that I should consume that dust.
➤ But the hedge of protection that you have place around Job won't allow me to do that!
➤ Not fair!

The picture the Bible is painting for us should be clear. *Ha satan* is the principality (principle enforcer) that is prowling the earth, "roaring like a lion, seeking whom he may devour" (1 Peter 5:8). But he is having a hard time devouring Job! By all accounts, Job should be denying God and showing deference to the dust of his constitution (Job 2:9). But he is not. He is stubbornly continuing to show deference to God, in spite of everything that the devil keeps throwing at him.

## The Great Testing

Writ large in the Bible is the great spiritual testing that we all face in a universe such as this. Let us ignore for the moment everything we have been saying about humankind's spiritual struggle against "increasing entropy," and focus instead on the metaphoric way in which the Bible describes the ordeal in the Book of Job. God has given the devil a charge over the *physical* constitution of man. God has not given the devil a charge over the *spiritual* constitution of man (Job 1:12). Not willing to exact his pound of flesh from Job's physical constitution, *ha satan* wants his pound of flesh from Job's spiritual constitution as well. As the Bible skillfully lets it be known, this is what *ha satan* wants from all of us, including you, dear reader (refer to Ephesians 6:11, Hebrews 2:14, James 4:7, 1 Peter 5:8).

Given that God made us from the physics of the universe (Genesis 2:7), the proverbial devil may be entitled to the pound of flesh that he exacts from our *physical* constitution—we must all grow old and eventually revert back to the stability of dust. Howbeit this devil is not entitled to the pound of flesh that he would exact from our *spiritual* constitution as well. That is, unless we, by our own default, sanction, and consent, allow him to do that. This, then, is the great contention of the Bible, the great testing ("great tribulation") that we all face in a universe in which life is a fugitive searching for the sanctuary of the Kingdom of God, by and by not finding it, even though it is very near to each and every one of us (Luke 17:21).

## The Love of God

Here and elsewhere, God reveals the desire of His heart to us. Our Heavenly Father wants us to love Him "in spirit and in truth" (John 4:23–24). Mind you, not because He is in need of veneration, but because He wants his children to remain spiritually whole, in spite of every effort of *ha satan* to the contrary. The creator of the universe wants real devotion from His children, because anything less would make His children prey to the devil's stratagems. God wants real commitment from us and will not settle for anything less. Throughout the Bible, our Heavenly Father makes it clear that He will not tolerate feigned commitment and lip service. He abhors lip service and has said so:

Hypocrites! Well did Isaiah prophesy about you, saying:

> "These people draw near to Me with their mouth,
> And honor Me with their lips,
> But their heart is far from Me.
> And in vain they worship Me,
> Teaching as doctrines the commandments of men."
> (Jesus Christ quoting Isaiah 29:13 in Matthew 15:7–9)

Job's affection, love, and reverence for God was the real thing, exactly what our Heavenly Father wants from all of us. Job was not obeying God in order to get something in return. He was obeying God because he loved God with all his heart, all his soul, and all his mind, per the great commandment found in Deuteronomy 6:5, echoed by Jesus Christ in Matthew 22:35–40:

> Then one of the Pharisees, a lawyer, asked Him a question, testing Him, and saying, "Teacher, which is the great commandment in the law?" Jesus said to him, "'You shall love the Lord your God with all your heart, with all your soul, and with all your mind.' This is the first and great commandment. And the second is like it: 'You shall love your neighbor as yourself.' On these two commandments hang all the Law and the Prophets."

## The Temptation in the Wilderness

I see you sitting on a church pew and shaking your head. I hear you say, "If the devil of the Bible is not a person, how then do you explain the temptation in the wilderness?" Let us bear in mind that Christ was alone in the wilderness. There was no CNN crew there to film the event! Meaning what? Meaning, the disciples must have learned of it through Jesus himself. Meaning, we must lay aside the superstitions that so easily distract and focus on what Christ is teaching us:

And the devil said to Him, "If You are the Son of God, command this stone to become bread." But Jesus answered him, saying, "It is written, 'Man shall not live by bread alone, but by every word of God.'" (Luke 4:3–4)

A great teaching! God does not deny our need for bread. Bread is good. Bread is necessary. "Bread" provides the food and sustenance that our bodies need to remain viable in a universe such as this. But we must never allow mere "bread" to become the be-all and end-all of our existence. As image bearers of God, there is much more to our existence than mere "bread" (matter and energy). The great truth that Christ is conveying to us here can be found throughout the syntactical whole of the Bible. The same truth that is being echoed by the Apostle Paul in his letter to the formative church in Rome:

> For the kingdom of God is not eating and drinking, but righteousness and peace and joy in the Holy Spirit. (Romans 14:17)

We say again: God has given the devil a charge over the rudiments of the perishable universe (matter and energy, aka food and drink). God has not given the devil a charge over the spiritual soul of humanity.

> Then the devil, taking Him up on a high mountain, showed Him all the kingdoms of the world in a moment of time. And the devil said to Him, "All this authority I will give You, and their glory; for this has been delivered to me, and I give it to whomever I wish. Therefore, if You will worship before me, all will be Yours." (Luke 4:5–7)

> And Jesus answered and said to him, "Get behind Me, Satan! For it is written, 'You shall worship the Lord your God, and Him only you shall serve.'" (Luke 4: 5–8)

Another great teaching! At all times and in all places, we are to give the primacy to the Creator and only relative subordinacy to the created thing.

At all times, and in all places, we must resist the temptation to worship the created thing instead of the Creator. As the Apostle Paul also cautions:

> Finally, my brethren, be strong in the Lord and in the power of His might. Put on the whole armor of God, that you may be able to stand against the wiles of the devil. For we do not wrestle against flesh and blood, but against principalities [Greek *archas*], against powers [Greek *exousias*], against the rulers [Greek *kosmocratoras*] of the darkness of this age, against spiritual hosts of wickedness in the heavenly places. (Ephesians 6:10-12)

## Ephesians 6:10–12

Most Christians would interpret Ephesians 6:10–12 through Manichaean lenses, assuming that the Greek terms *archas, exousias,* and *kosmocratoras* refer to devils, demons, poltergeists, and diabolical entities. The truth may be much simpler than that, as indeed the truth often is. The Greek term *arché*, for example (Strong's Greek 746) translated "principalities," hails from a primitive verb implying "beginning, original, chief, fundamental, primary, princely, principle, pre-existing, predominant in categories of space, time, nature, necessity, rank, and authority." From this root, we derive words such as *archaic, archangel, archbishop, archduke, archetype, archetypal, architect, archive,* and *archivist.* The Oxford Companion to Philosophy has this to say about the Greek term *arché*:

> A first thing from which something is, or comes to be, or is known ... Applied to materials which do not arise out of anything more primitive, to causes of change, to propositions fundamental in deductive systems, by teleologists to benefits and beneficiaries, and, colloquially, since they are sources of initiates in states, to governments.[39]

The Greek term translated *power* in Ephesians 6:12 is *exousia* (Strong's

---

[39] *The Oxford Companion to Philosophy,* edited by Ted Honderich (New York: Oxford University Press, 1995) 58.

Greek 1849), which many versions of the Bible render "authority." Elsewhere, the Bible uses the term to refer to governmental authorities:

> Let every soul be subject to the governing authorities [<Greek, *exousia*]. For there is no authority [<Greek, *exousia*] except from God, and the authorities [<Greek, *exousia*] that exist are appointed by God. (Romans 13:1)

Straining Ephesians 6:12 through Manichaean filters would have us believe that God had elevated devils and demons to the status of governing authorities, an absurd notion contrary to the habit and practice of Christ in casting them out. The Greek term translated *rulers of the darkness of this age* in Ephesians 6:12 is *kosmocratoras* (Strong's Greek 2888), signifying "world dictators," at that time typified by godless, brutal, satanic emperors like Nero and Caligula.

Forcing the Bible by the rules of a Manichaean worldview does not help the cause of Christ, dear friends. It makes the Christian Church the laughingstock of the whole world.

## Will the Real Devil Please Stand Up!

Is there equivalence between the personal Manichaean devil that most Christians believe in, and the impersonal Augustinian devil that most have never even heard of? At first glance, you'd think that there was. Whatever you might say about the Manichaean devil, for example, the same could be said of the Augustinian devil. Both devils are principalities (principle enforcers). Both discriminate against the unstable complexity of life, the former deterministically, the latter statistically. If the Manichaean devil is out to destroy life, so is the Augustinian devil. If the Manichaean devil is out to destroy structure, so is the Augustinian devil. If the Manichaean devil is out to reduce the unstable complexity of life to the stability of simple dust, so is Augustinian devil. On the face of it, at least, you'd think that there was equivalence between the two. But there is not. The two devils differ in one major way. The personal Manichaean devil that most Christians believe in can only be in one place at a time, whereas the impersonal Augustinian devil can be in all places simultaneously. This poses a serious problem for those who continue to believe in a personal devil called "Lucifer." Case in point:

> Then Satan entered Judas, surnamed Iscariot, who was numbered among the twelve. So he went his way and conferred with the chief priests and captains, how he might betray Him [Jesus] to them. And they were glad, and agreed to give him money. So he promised and sought opportunity to betray Him to them in the absence of the multitude. (Luke 22:3–6)

Clearly, "Lucifer" can only be in one place at a time, here, for example, in the body of Judas, elsewhere in the bodies of Hitler, or Stalin, or some such *kosmokrator* (dictator). What are we to think? When "Lucifer" was preoccupied with possessing the body of Judas the remainder of humanity was being spared his predations? How does that square with the testimony of the Bible? Well, if the Bible is clear about one thing, it is that "all have sinned and come short of the glory of God" (Romans 3:23). What then? In that *all* have sinned, *all* must have been *personally* tempted, deceived, and corrupted by "Lucifer"? What's wrong with this picture?

There is contradiction between the Manichaean devil that most Christians were brought up to believe in, and the Augustinian devil that the Bible calls *ha satan*. The two are not compatible. There is no equivalence between the two. There is, however, strong equivalence between the devil that the Bible calls *ha satan* and the principality that we have been calling "Cosmic Constable" throughout this publication. Certainly, a principality (principle enforcer) that discriminates against life, structure, and complexity would correspond with the principality that Christ alludes to:

> The thief does not come except to steal, and to kill, and to destroy. I have come that they may have life, and that they may have it more abundantly. (John 10:10)

If you have been following the discourse of this publication, you should have no trouble correlating the words of Christ with the modus operandi of the principality we have been calling "Cosmic Constable." Certainly, this "Cosmic Constable" could be said to be the great *antagonist* of life, structure, and complexity; the great *protagonist* of nonlife, non-structure, and simplicity. Naturally, the transition from life to nonlife could involve "killing." Naturally, the transition from structure to non-structure could involve "de-struction." No doubt about it; the Cosmic Constable "comes to steal, and to kill, and to destroy."

So then, if there is strong equivalence between the devil of the Bible and the principality that we have been calling "Cosmic Constable," we may have uncovered a bane much larger than "cancer" in this epic journey of ours. We may have laid bare the motives that underwrite the anatomy of human destructiveness. Let us not boast, however, as though we had discovered something new. Thousands of years before the advent of modern science the Bible was describing that same bane in this way:

> There is a way which seems right unto a man, but the end
> thereof are the ways of death.
> (Proverbs 14:12)

# Index

www.ingramcontent.com/pod-product-compliance
Lightning Source LLC
Chambersburg PA
CBHW051447250726

48655CB00001B/275